D1234259

The Maillard Reaction

The Maillard Reaction

Consequences for the Chemical and Life Sciences

Edited by

RAPHAEL IKAN

Hebrew University of Jerusalem, Israel

JOHN WILEY & SONS

Chichester · New York · Brisbane · Toronto · Singapore

Other Wiley Editorial Offices

John Wiley & Sons, Inc., 605 Third Avenue,
New York, NY 10158-0012, USA

Jacaranda Wiley Ltd, 33 Park Road, Milton,
Queensland 4064, Australia

John Wiley & Sons (Canada) Ltd, 22 Worcester Road,
Rexdale, Ontario M9W 1L1, Canada

John Wiley & Sons (SEA) Pte Ltd, 2 Clementi Loop #02-01,
Jin Xing Distripark, Singapore 0512

British Library Cataloguing in Publication Data

A catalogue record for this book is available from the British Library

ISBN 0-471-96300-3

Typeset in 10/12pt Times by Dobbie Typesetting Ltd
Printed and bound in Great Britain by Bookcraft (Bath) Ltd

This book is printed on acid-free paper responsibly manufactured from sustainable forestation,
for which at least two trees are planted for each one used for paper production.

To my wife, Yael, and our favorite offspring,
who enjoy her tasty Maillard-flavored food.

Contents

List of Contributors

PROFESSOR JOHN W. BAYNES

Department of Chemistry and Biochemistry and School of Medicine, University of South Carolina, Columbia, SC 29208, USA

PROFESSOR RICHARD BUCALA

The Picower Institute for Medical Research, 350 Community Drive, Manhasset, NY 11030, USA

PROFESSOR ANTHONY CERAMI

The Picower Institute for Medical Research, 350 Community Drive, Manhasset, NY 11030, USA

DR MENDEL FRIEDMAN

USDA-ARS, Western Regional Research Center, 800 · Buchanan Street, Albany, CA 94710, USA

PROFESSOR F. HAYASE

Department of Agricultural Chemistry, Meiji University, 1-1-1 Higashi-mita, Tama-ku, Kawasaki, Kanagawa 214, Japan

PROFESSOR CHI-TANG HO

Department of Food Science, Rutgers State University, PO Box 231, New Brunswick, NJ 08903-0231, USA

PROFESSOR RAPHAEL IKAN

Department of Organic Chemistry, Hebrew University of Jerusalem, Jerusalem 91904, Israel

PROFESSOR I. R. KAPLAN

Institute of Geophysics and Planetary Physics, University of California Los Angeles, USA

PROFESSOR A. NISSENBAUM

Weizmann Institute of Science, Rehovot, Israel

PROFESSOR TAKAYUKI SHIBAMOTO

Department of Environmental Toxicology, University of California Davis, Davis, CA 95616, USA

DR Y. RUBINSZTAIN

Department of Organic Chemistry, Hebrew University of Jerusalem, Jerusalem 91904, Israel

PROFESSOR SIMON P. WOLFF

Formerly of *Toxicology Laboratory, Department of Medicine, University College London Medical School, London WC1E 6JJ, England*

DR JON W. WONG

Department of Environmental Toxicology, University of California Davis, Davis, CA 95616, USA

PROFESSOR V. A. YAYLAYAN

Department of Food Science and Agricultural Chemistry, McGill University, 2111 Lakeshore Road, Ste Anne de Bellevue, Quebec, Canada H9X 3V9

Preface

The term Maillard reaction, or nonenzymatic browning, was coined in honor of its inventor, Louis-Camille Maillard. It is related to the reaction between amines and carbonyl compounds, especially reducing sugars. It has been detected in heated, dried or stored foods and in the mammalian organisms. In food stuffs, the Maillard reaction is responsible for changes in the flavor, color, nutritive value and the formation of mutagenic compounds. *In vivo* aging and the complications of diabetes are partly ascribed to the interaction of glucose and proteins.

Mauron has divided the Maillard reaction into three stages: early, advanced and final. The first corresponds to the chemically well-defined stages, without browning (flavors, etc.), and the second to the innumerable reactions leading to the final stage of formation of insoluble brown polymers (melanoidins). Maillard reactions are strongly dependent on the reaction conditions. The most important parameters are duration and temperature of heating, moisture content, pH and type of sugar present.

This book tries to show the present state of the art in the development of new horizons and approaches of the Maillard reactions in the following topics: the Maillard reaction under physiological conditions, its impact on aging, its anticarcinogenic effects, free radicals and glycation theory, genotoxicity, generation of aromas, the effect on nutritional values of food, nonenzymatic glycation, geochemical aspects, DNA cleavage of glycated proteins, biological recognition of Maillard reaction products, scavenging of active oxygens and microwave-induced Maillard reaction.

The wealth of information presented in this book by well-known scientists on the multidisciplinary nature of the Maillard reaction may open up the way for a cross-fertilization between the various disciplines.

Although this book cannot give a complete account of the Maillard reaction, we hope that it will furnish important information on its various aspects. The Maillard reaction is regarded as a 'simple' and an easy reaction to carry out in the laboratory; however, the mechanism of this reaction is rather complex.

Furthermore, its involvement in many interdisciplinary fields is remarkable. In this respect it is incomparable to any other chemical reaction.

This book might be of interest to scientists engaged in research in the following areas: biochemistry, biology, chemistry, geochemistry, nutrition, food, physiology, toxicology and other areas.

I would like to take this opportunity to express my gratitude to the contributing authors and the publisher.

Raphael Ikan
Department of Organic Chemistry,
Laboratory of Natural Products and
Organic Geochemistry, Hebrew University of
Jerusalem, Israel and
The Institute of Geophysics and
Planetary Physics, University of California
Los Angeles (UCLA), USA

List of Abbreviations

AGE	Advanced Glycosylation End-products
BSA	Bovin Serum Albumin
^{13}C-CP-MAS NMR	^{13}C-Cross Polarized Magic Angle Spinning Nuclear Magnetic Resonance
CML	Carboxymethyllysine
EDTA	Ethylene Diamine Tetra Acetate
ESR	Electron Spin Resonance
FFI	Furoyl Furanyl Imidazole
GC-MS	Gas Chromatography-Mass Spectrometry
HHA	Heterocyclic Aromatic Amines
HPLC	High Performance Liquid Chromatography
HS	Humic Substances
LC-MS	Liquid Chromatography-Mass Spectrum
LDL	Low Density Lipoproteins
MRP	Maillard Reaction Products
NFP	Novel Fluorophore
NMR	Nuclear Magnetic Resonance
NPR	Net Protein Ratio
NPU	Net Protein Utilization
PER	Protein Efficiency Ratio
PNV	Protein Nutritional Value
UV	Ultra Violet

1

Geochemical Aspects of the Maillard Reaction

R. IKAN[1], Y. RUBINSZTAIN[1], A. NISSENBAUM[2]
and I. R. KAPLAN[3]

[1]Department of Organic Chemistry, Hebrew University of Jerusalem, Israel
[2]Weizmann Institute of Science, Rehovot, Israel
[3]Institute of Geophysics and Planetary Physics,
University of California Los Angeles, USA

Brown acidic polymers known as humic substances account for much of the organic material that occurs in soils, natural waters and recent sediments (Borkovsky, 1965). It has long been recognized that the degradation products of lignin can react with proteins and amino acids to form humic substances (Flaig, 1964). Since the work of Maillard (1913), evidence has accumulated which suggests that natural humic substances may also be produced by condensation reactions between sugars and amino acids (Enders and Theis, 1938; Hodge, 1953; Abelson and Hare, 1971). This evidence is based upon chemical similarities between natural humic substances and sugar–amino acid condensation products (melanoidins) produced in the laboratory (Hoering, 1973) and upon the occurrence of indigenous humic substances in marine environments, where carbohydrates and proteins or their degradation products, because of their abundance, are more likely precursors of humic substances than are lignin polymers (Nissenbaum and Kaplan, 1972; Hedges and Parker, 1976). Ertel and Hedges (1983) as well as Ikan et al. (1986a) have tested the hypothesis that marine (and also possibly terrestrial) humic acids contain a quantitatively significant melanoidin component. The experimental approach of the two groups was to compare the chemical and spectroscopic characteristics of representative marine and terrestrial humic acids with each

The Maillard Reaction: Consequences for the Clinical and Life Sciences. Edited by Raphael Ikan
©1996 John Wiley & Sons Ltd

Table 1.1. Elemental composition data for melanoidins (SG = sugar, AA = amino acid, Exp. = expected, Det. = determined). (Reprinted with permission from R. Ikan, T. Dorsey and I. R. Kaplan, *Anal. Chim. Acta*, **232**, 11, 1990. Copyright 1990, Elsevier Science)

Number	Melanoidin (SG–AA)	Molar ratio	Elemental analysis (%)						Atomic ratio					
			Exp. C	Det. C	Exp. H	Det. H	Exp. N	Det. N	Exp. N/C	Det. N/C	Exp. H/C	Det. H/C	Exp. O/C	Det. O/C
1	Glu–Lys	9:1	57.28	59.50	5.54	7.25	2.26	4.00	0.034	0.060	1.15	1.21	0.458	0.48
2	Glu–Tyr	9:1	58.53	55.23	5.15	4.99	1.10	2.36	0.016	0.037	1.05	1.08	0.452	0.43
3	Glu–Net	9:1	59.28	57.24	5.22	5.53	1.12	2.70	0.016	0.041	1.05	1.16	0.435	0.41
4	Gal:Iso	9:1	57.98	58.96	5.53	5.72	1.15	2.16	0.017	0.033	1.14	1.14	0.458	0.51
5	Gal:Gly	9:1	56.65	55.08	5.10	5.23	1.20	2.15	0.018	0.022	1.07	1.18	0.491	0.49
6	Glu–Val	9:1	57.66	59.86	5.42	4.75	1.16	1.50	0.017	0.030	1.12	1.15	0.466	0.46
7	Gal–Asp	9:1	56.99	57.44	5.21	5.51	1.19	2.02	0.018	0.030	1.09	1.25	0.482	0.50
8	Gal–Lys	9:1	57.28	53.83	5.54	5.65	2.26	4.47	0.034	0.071	1.15	1.85	0.458	0.49
9	Gal–Lys	1:1	57.87	56.63	8.83	6.71	12.27	9.03	0.182	0.159	1.82	1.34	0.273	0.49
10	Glu–Lys	1:1	57.87	51.92	8.83	5.80	12.27	8.11	0.182	0.130	1.82	1.06	0.273	0.46
11	Glu–Tyr	1:1	63.86	53.99	6.51	5.35	5.32	3.28	0.071	0.056	1.21	1.18	0.286	0.42
12	Gal–Gly	1:1	53.49	45.59	7.05	5.27	8.91	6.72	0.143	0.052	1.57	1.26	0.429	0.35
13	Gal–Iso	1:1	61.94	60.07	8.98	6.28	6.57	5.52	0.091	0.079	1.73	1.43	0.273	0.44
14	Glu–Val	1:1	60.28	56.08	8.60	6.66	7.03	4.51	0.100	0.069	1.70	1.17	0.300	0.63
15	Glu–Cys	1:1	56.12	41.93	7.65	4.09	8.18	6.00	0.125	0.122	1.63	0.99	0.375	0.45
16	Glu–Asp	1:1	56.12	56.37	7.65	4.63	8.18	4.83	0.125	0.073	1.63	1.58	0.375	0.63
17	Glu–Lys	1:9	58.57	45.15	12.72	5.93	24.11	10.47	0.353	0.200	2.59	1.58	0.059	0.63
18	Gal–Lys	1:9	58.57	51.61	12.72	6.80	24.11	5.33	0.353	0.193	2.59	1.58	0.059	0.63
19	Gal–Gly	1:9	44.41	37.59	12.67	4.36	31.08	6.87	0.600	0.156	3.40	1.39	0.200	1.02
20	Gal–Val	1:9	64.31	59.61	13.49	7.85	16.08	10.21	0.214	0.170	2.50	1.31	0.071	0.37
21	Glu–Cys	1:9	54.19	37.72	13.08	7.04	23.71	5.10	0.375	0.185	2.88	1.56	0.071	0.49
22	Glu–Tyr	1:9	68.84	51.40	7.78	5.01	9.27	3.65	0.154	0.061	1.35	1.16	0.125	0.70
23	Gal–Lys	1:19	58.67	43.95	13.26	5.73	25.75	9.50	0.376	0.120	2.69	1.34	0.115	0.37
24	Glu–Ala	1:1	56.12	57.38	7.65	6.43	8.18	7.81	0.125	0.090	1.63	0.99	0.030	0.58
25	Glu–Ala	1:1	56.12	51.25	7.65	4.69	8.18	4.25	0.125	0.090	1.63	1.08	0.375	0.40

Glu = glucose; Ala = alanine; Asp = aspartic acid; Cys = cystine; Gal = galactose; Gly = glycine; Iso = isoleucine; Lys = lysine; Met = methionine; Tyr = tyrosine; Val = valine.

other and with parallel suites of 'phenolic' melanoidin synthesized in the laboratory under controlled conditions from sugars and amino acids. The synthetic polymers of Ertel and Hedges were produced by reacting either glucose (hypothesized marine pathway) or catechol (hypothesized terrestrial pathway) with either ammonia or the amino acid alanine, and Rubinsztain *et al.* (1984) reacted glucose or galactose with various amino acids which represent major forms of nitrogenous substances found in natural environments that are apparently involved in humic acid formation. Although possibly an oversimplification, synthetic humic acids (melanoidins) provide a means of recognizing compositional characteristics that are precursor related. In addition, the effects of reactant ratios, reaction conditions and the extent of reaction on these characteristics can be systematically determined and compared. Comparatively little structural information has been reported for melanoidins. Ertel and Hedges (1983) have analyzed the synthetic polymers (melanoidins) and representative marine and terrestrial humic acids for their elemental compositions and IR, UV, fluorescence and electron spin resonance spectroscopic properties. They claim that synthetic humic acids have elemental and spectroscopic properties generally similar to the natural geopolymers. The melanoidins most closely resemble the marine humic acids, whereas the synthetic phenolic polymers resemble the terrestrial humic acids. They did not suggest, however, any structural formulae.

The various opinions expressed by scientists concerning chemical structural aspects and chemical behavior of melanoidins started by Maillard in 1912 are still being investigated today (Mauron, 1981; Olsson *et al.*, 1981; Hayase and Kato, 1981). Unfortunately, each research group synthesized the melanoidins under different conditions using different reactants.

In order to gain more structural information Rubinsztain *et al.* (1984) have synthesized various series of melanoidins by using different ratios (mostly 9:1, 1:9 and 1:1) of sugars and amino acids. The synthetic melanoidins (in alkaline solution) were subjected to a variety of spectroscopic (IR, ^{13}C-CP-MAS NMR), destructive (pyrolysis, oxidation) and nondestructive (ESR) methods. This approach has provided a wealth of information on melanoidins derived from the *same* amino acids and sugars. In some cases, e.g. Gal–Ileu and Gal–Arg (Gal = galactose, Ileu = isoleucine, Arg = arginine), more than one melanoidin was isolated. Some of the melanoidins formed precipitated during the synthesis, whereas in most cases the dark brown solution was clear. The yields were sugar dependent. Under the same reaction conditions glucose and galatose (with no amino acid) formed a 'melanoidin-like' polymer (pseudomelanoidin), indicating that reducing sugars can 'caramelize' under mild conditions (100 °C), not only at high (> 250–400 °C) temperatures. The elementary analysis of some melanoidins is summarized in Table 1.1. This table reveals the following trends: (a) the nitrogen content depends on the type of amino acid (AA) and sugar (SG) ratio; (b) the N/C atomic ratio reflects the

SG/AA ratio; (c) the H/C ratio does not reflect only CH bonds but rather heteroatom-bonded hydrogen (mostly oxygen); (d) the O/C ratio is relatively constant; (e) the galactose polymer indicates the loss of 3 H_2O units. The loss of CO_2 is due to amino acid decarboxylation. Gel filtration molecular weight analysis reveals that the molecular weight of most samples is above 10 000 m.w.u. (molecular weight units). The galactose–lysine (1 : 1) sample exhibited the highest m.w.u. value of $\geqslant 20\,000$. Using the ultracentrifugation technique the molecular weight of some of the melanoidins was in the range of 10 000–30 000 m.w.u. The fact that the m.w.u. melanoidins of the basic amino acids and sugars are higher than those prepared from neutral and acidic amino acids indicates the probability of cross-linking. This was supported by the thermal stability study (DTG). The 'fulvic' and 'humic' properties of melanoidins probably stem from their acidic character.

Acidic determination of melanoidins revealed that the 'overall' acidity stems mostly from the sugar moiety; the carboxylic group contributes up to 20% of the total acidity (Table 1.2). It seems that the carboxyl acidity is correlated with the relative contribution of sugar; the higher the SG/AA ratio, the higher is the carboxyl group concentration. The IR study of Gal–Gly (glycine) (9 : 1) melanoidin shows the $1705\,\text{cm}^{-1}$ absorbance of the COOH. Peaks at 1380 and $1610\,\text{cm}^{-1}$ are due to COO^- and are attributed to furanyl ring vibrations as well as the 1370 and $1025\,\text{cm}^{-1}$ bands. None of the melanoidins had an amide absorbance.

In an attempt to follow the kinetics of melanoidin formation the UV–VIS spectra were monitored (270 nm) in a special ambient trap to imitate natural conditions using glucose–lysine (1 : 1). A very slow reaction occurred at 25 °C,

Table 1.2. Acidity values for selected melanoidin samples and comparison with humic acids. (Reprinted with permission from Y. Rubinsztain, P. Ioselis, R. Ikan and Z. Aizenshtat, *Organic Geochemistry*, **6**, 804, 1984. Copyright 1984, Elsevier Science Ltd)

Melanoidin (ratio)	Total acidity (meq/g)	Carboxylic acidity (meq/g)	Phenolic acidity (meq/g)
Gal	12.28	1.79	10.49
Gal–Lys (9 : 1)	11.41		
Gal–Lys (1 : 1)	6.23		
Gal–Gly (9 : 1)	8.52	2.07	6.45
Gal–Ileu 'A' (9 : 1)	12.45	2.30	10.15
Gal–Ileu (9 : 1)	9.03	1.43	7.60
Gal–Ileu (1 : 1)	8.38	1.48	6.90
Gal–Ileu (1 : 9)	6.86	1.22	5.64
Gal–Val (9 : 1)	12.44		
Gal–Glu acid (9 : 1)	13.63	2.61	11.02
Gal–Glu acid 'H' (9 : 1)	11.91	2.68	9.23
Humic acid	8.93	4.10	4.83

whereas elevation of the temperature to 55 or 75 °C changes the reaction rate dramatically. A set of experiments was left at room temperature for 4 years and from the intensity of the color it appears that the higher the SG/AA ratio, the more melanoidin is formed. The kinetics and yield of melanoidin synthesis depends on temperature and availability of the sugar.

In order to obtain structural information of humic substances, several *oxidation methods* have been used: $KMnO_4$ (Schnitzer, 1977; Ogner, 1973; Machihara and Ishiwatari, 1983), cupric oxide (Schnitzer and de Serra, 1973) in alkaline media and persulfate oxidation (Martin *et al.*, 1981). Ishiwatari *et al.* (1986) have found that the relative abundance and the relative amounts of benzene di-, tri- and tetracarboxylic acids from lake Karuna humin resembles those of the melanoidins and pseudomelanoidins. It appears, therefore, that a significant portion of the lake sedimentary humin is contributed by melanoidins and/or pseudomelanoidins, although the extent of their contribution is yet unknown.

Recent developments in the NMR spectroscopy of solids has demonstrated the advantage of using a combined *NMR cross-polarization technique* which enhances sensitivity and high power protein decoupling, thus decreasing line broadening (Pugmire *et al.*, 1982; Hatcher *et al.*, 1980a, 1980b). Further elimination in line broadening is achieved by spinning the sample at high speed so that the axis is oriented at a magic angle (54.7°) with respect to the external magnetic field (Andrew, 1972). The combined technique (CP-MAS) results in high-resolution spectra and enables structure elucidation of complex fossil fuels.

It has been observed (Ikan *et al.*, 1986b) that the AAM-type melanoidins possess aliphatic resonances of the original amino acids, including α-carbons. The survival of the peak at 55 ppm (of Gal–Lys, 9:1 melanoidin) after acid hydrolysis and dipolar dephasing indicates the presence of a nonprotonated C-2 atom (carbon adjacent to nitrogen), probably as R_3C-N protonated bond.

The participation of amino acids such as lysine and isoleucine in the melanoidin synthesis increases the formation of the aliphatic fraction up to 50% of the total carbons of melanoidins. The presence of aliphatic moieties in humic substances was revealed by NMR spectra by Gonzalez Vila *et al.* (1976), Ogner (1979) and Wilson and Goh (1977). Recently, Hatcher *et al.* (1980a, 1980b, 1981) have recorded the presence of relatively large quantities of aliphatics both in marine and terrestrial environments.

The resemblance of NMR peaks of HHA (hula humic acid) and melanoidins which were synthesized from lysine (Rubinsztain *et al.*, 1984) might be due to fast reaction of lysine with reducing sugar (Hedges, 1978) and the dominance of lysine in hula peat. The split peak at 70–76 ppm is present in most melanoidins and HHA and is due to protonated α-carbon which is linked to an oxygenated carbon of polysaccharides (Preston and Schnitzer, 1984; Wilson *et al.*, 1981). The peak at 62 ppm of the AAM-type melanoidin (Gal–Ileu, 1:9) probably corresponds to a protonated α-carbon atom which is linked to the nitrogen atom of isoleucine.

The peak of 70–76 ppm is present in Gal–Iso (1 : 9) melanoidin and probably confirms its hydrophilic character. The band at 60–65 ppm is probably due to a primary alcohol group (Mikita *et al.*, 1981). The strong band at 58 ppm may be assigned as methoxyl or ether bonded aliphatic carbon or aliphatic OH (Dereppe *et al.*, 1980; Gonzales Vila *et al.*, 1983).

The high resonance signal in the aromatic region might be due to the carbons forming the polymeric core of the melanoidins. The broad absorption in the 132–135 ppm region might be due to the conjugation of olefinic moieties with furanoids or aromatic rings (Benzing-Purdie *et al.*, 1985). The band in the 105–160 ppm region might also be due to the different heterocyclic moieties, some of which are known to be formed by the Maillard reaction. The formation of these compounds is highly influenced by acid/base conditions (Shaw *et al.*, 1968; Hicks and Feather, 1975). It has been reported (Wolfrom *et al.*, 1947; Hodge, 1953) that sugars under alkaline conditions and in the presence of amino acids enolize and form amino reductons and methylglyoxal. These active molecules as well as furanones, furfuryl alcohol and hydroxyl-cyclopentenones may polymerize by the catalytic effect of amino acids in weakly alkaline media (Chuang *et al.*, 1984; Hodge, 1953). Recently Gillam and Wilson (1985) reported the ^{13}C-CP-MAS NMR spectra of humic substances isolated from a coastal marine environment with a main peak in the aromatic region centered at 135–136 ppm, which remarkably resembles the resonance band (3) of our melanoidins (Figure 1.1).

We find that the ^{13}C-CP-MAS NMR spectra of melanoidins have a remarkable resemblance to some humic acids. Hence it is suggested that the Maillard reaction (of sugars and amino acids) plays a more significant role in the formation of the skeletal matrix structure of humic substances than previously thought.

ELECTRON SPIN RESONANCE

Free radicals of humic substances (HS) were extensively studied by ESR (EPR) spectroscopy. These studies indicated that the free radical density (Ng) of HS is usually in the range of 18^{18} spin/g (Steelink, 1964; Nissenbaum and Kaplan, 1972; Riffaldi and Schnitzer, 1972; Senesi and Schnitzer, 1977). Durand *et al.* (1977) have investigated the ESR signals of various types of kerogens as a function of the evolution stage. They found that a good correlation exists between natural and heat-treated kerogens. It has been suggested that the humic/melanoidin-type materials are the diagenetic precursors of kerogens. A correlative similarity should therefore exist between the ESR signals of the maturation sequence of the kerogens and the pyrolyzed humic/melanoidin

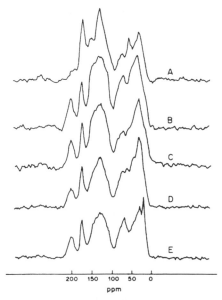

Figure 1.1. ^{13}C-CP/MAS NMR of SM-type melanoidins: A, hula humic acid (HAA); B, galactose–glucose (9:1); C, galactose–glycine (9:1); D, galactose–lysine (9:1); E, galactose–valine (9:1). (Reprinted with permission from R. Ikan, Y Rubinsztain, P. Ioselis, Z. Aizenshtat, R. Pugmire and L. L. Anderson, *Organic Geochemistry*, **9**, 199, 1986. Copyright 1986, Elsevier Science Ltd)

materials. This technique was applied for synthetic HS and melanoidins (Mathur and Schnitzer, 1978; Lessig and Bates, 1982; Ertel and Hedges, 1983; Aizenshtat *et al.*, 1987). The ESR measurements of stepwise-pyrolyzed melanoidins and HS (at various temperatures, mesh size and pH values) furnished the information shown in Table 1.3. The *g* and *Ng* values of melanoidins are similar to those of the HS, suggesting that the melanoidin structure stabilizes the long-lived free radicals in a manner similar to HS. Cleavage of $C-C$ and $C-X$ (X = heteroatom) bonds increases the *Ng* value. The authors concluded that the thermal behavior of melanoidins is in good correlation with that of type III kerogen (Tissot *et al.*, 1974).

Pyrolysis of humic substances and melanoidins in closed systems (autoclave or sealed ampoules) yielded a series of light hydrocarbons and volatile products. The yield of C-1–C-4 hydrocarbons obtained by pyrolysis of certain melanoidins was considerably higher than those obtained from HS. Pyrolysis of both HS and melanoidins produced sugar-derived products, mainly furan derivatives. In general the pyrolysis of melanoidins produced more oxygen-containing compounds than hydrocarbons, and only in the cases where the initial ratio of AA used in the preparation of melanoidins was dominant did an appreciable amount of hydrocarbons form (Table 1.4). Although the

Table 1.3. Free radicals density $(Ng)^a$ of thermally treated melanoidins and humic substances. (Reprinted with permission from Z. Aizenshtat, Y. Rubinsztain, P. Ioselis, I. Miloslavsky and R. Ikan, *Organic Geochemistry*, **11**, 65, 1987. Copyright 1984, Elsevier Science Ltd)

Melanoidin (ratio)	Temperature (°C)								
	100	150	200	250	300	350	400	450	500
Gal 200 mesh		2.40	7.26	28.16		165.10	95.71		33.51
Gal–Lys (9:1)	1.89	1.43		12.16	44.18	33.20	16.89	16.20	
Gal–Lys (9:1) 200 mesh	0.36		12.76		20.75		15.78		
Gal–Val (9:1)	1.62	1.75		23.12	62.78	28.00	18.72	11.21	
Gal–Val (9:1) 200 mesh	0.43		1.85		29.52		10.94		
Gal–Tyr (9:1)	1.62	1.69		48.87	56.49	35.18	23.46	26.28	
Gal–Tyr (9:1) 200 mesh	0.58		1.54		24.92		8.39		
Gal–bovine albumin		0.86	2.60	12.75	34.20	32.40	45.53		31.88
Gal–Arg 'A' (1:1) 200 mesh	0.60	1.40	2.72	3.20	6.11	5.05	10.40	130.90	77.80
Gal–Arg 200 mesh	0.17	1.34	2.01	1.65	4.60	9.30	39.70	53.50	67.10
Gal–Arg $(NH_4S_x^-)$ 200 mesh	0.30	0.60	0.80	2.60	5.90	8.90	36.20	86.60	116.40
HHa (hula humic acid)	0.39		4.17		5.30		5.06		
HHA 200 mesh	1.32	1.37		10.21	32.99	28.97	32.62	25.40	
Humic acid (Aldrich)	0.21		2.67		7.72		9.19		
Humic acid (Aldrich) 200 mesh	0.66	0.82		5.15	9.62	10.63	9 95	8.32	
HHA (6N HCl)	2.80	5.44	5.59	17.64	13.03				
HHA pH 6	1.38	4.50	5.74	11.36	28.34	81.86	65.00	37.58	
HHA pH 8	1.98	1.17	2.86	14.46	22.03	55.35	42.62	50.34	
HHA pH 10		5.10	14.50	32.20	71.25	87.28	70.60		45.48
HHA pH 10 + N_2		8.50	13.50	31.30	56.84	33.43	42.70		31.53

^{a}Number of free electrons per gram of sample.

laboratory-synthesized melanoidins do not consititute a proof that melanoidins are necessary for HS formation, they do add evidence that melanoidin-like polymers may compose a substantial component of the total humic material occurring in marine environments and in other locations where lignin degradation products are not prevalent.

ISOTOPIC ANALYSES

Humic acids extracted from *marine* sediments have $\delta^{13}C$ values typical of marine plankton, suggesting that the bulk carbon is autochthonous. The

Table 1.4. Hydrocarbons (C-1–C-4) formed by heat treatment of organic matter up to 350 °C (μg/g organic matter). (Reprinted with permission from R. Ikan, P. Ioselis, Y. Rubinsztain, Z. Aizenshtat, M. Muller-Vonmoos and A. Rub, *Organic Geochemistry*, **12**, 272, 1988. Copyright 1988, Elsevier Science Ltd)

Gas	Sample									
	M-2	M-3/Al$_2$O$_3$	M-3	HHA/Al$_2$O$_3$	HHA	HFA/Al$_2$O$_3$	Staten[a] post	Algal[a] mat	Tanner[a] Basin	Duck[a] Lake
Methane	5230	2080	3480	2040	2670	910	1280	2000	25800	5940
Ethene	1580	430	600	400	380	580	450	710	1130	1770
Ethane	10270	1560	2730	1070	1250	360	900	2060	9540	4880
Propene	3080	3760	1670	1880	700	3450	320	2720	1700	2900
Propane	7550	2470	4350	890	1270	310	680	2460	4780	3280
Isobutane	207	1700	3230	130	250	50	180	1200	1420	660
1-Butene (isobutene)	1960	2000	5060	470	930	610	550	4820	1040	1970
2-Butene (*trans*) (n-Butane)	5910	500	—	470	670	350	290[b]	1310[b]	250[b]	1030[b]
2-Butene (*cis*)	900	270	—	220	90	550	50[b]	760[b]	260[b]	480[b]
Hydrocarbons (total)	36690	14770	21120	7570	8210	7200	4600	18030	45900	22900
Ethene/ethane	0.15	0.27	0.22	0.37	0.30	1.6	0.50	0.34	0.12	0.36
Propene/propane	0.41	1.52	0.38	2.10	0.55	11.1	0.47	1.10	0.35	0.88
G1/C-1-C-4	0.14	0.14	0.16	0.27	0.32	0.13	0.28	0.11	0.56	0.26

[a] n-Butane. For M-2 mixed with Al$_2$O$_3$, the ethene/ethane ratio was 1.6 and the propene/propane ratio 5.1.
[b] 2-Butene. M-2 = galactose–lysine, 1:1; M-3 = galactose–valine, 9:1.

terrestrial humic acids show a characteristic wide range of $\delta^{13}C$ values, depending on whether they are derived from C^{-3} or C^{-4} plants.

Humic acids comprise a major part of the organic carbon reservoir in near-shore marine sediments. Marine humic substances fall in the range of $\delta^{13}C = -22\%$. The carbon isotope data suggest that the primary highly oxygenated polymer (*gelbstoff*) is transformed first into fulvic acid type compounds as intermediates in humification. The fulvic acids are isotopically close to the $\delta^{13}C$ values for plankton and are depleted in ^{13}C as compared with the humic acids.

During the transformation of fulvic into humic acids the condensation reaction is accompanied by loss of ^{13}C-enriched moieties. The synthetic humic substances (melanoidins) are regarded as closely related to marine humic substances. The stable carbon isotopic composition of melanoidin synthesized by Engel *et al.* (1986) indicated that it was depleted in carbon-13 as compared to the initial mixture of the starting materials (glucose and amino acids), especially of histidine. Engel *et al.* (1986) have pointed out that the mechanism that may be responsible for the ^{13}C depletion of the melanoidin relative to the starting materials could be due to the decarboxylation of amino acids via the Strecker degradation, occurring during the melanoidin formation (Hodge, 1953). A similar mechanism was suggested by Nissenbaum (1973) regarding the formation of melanoidins in the marine environment (via the condensation of amino acids and sugars). The possible 'generic' relationship between the marine humic acids and the melanoidins is supported by the stable carbon isotopic data of the two entities, as confirmed by a recent work of Ikan *et al.* (1990) on stable carbon and nitrogen isotopes of natural and synthetic humic substances (melanoidins). The isotope data of selected melanoidins and humic substances are summarized in Table 1.5.

The stable isotopic data presented in the table are in accordance with elemental composition data. These findings support assertions regarding the mechanism of the melanoidin reaction and its participation in the formation of marine humic substances. They indicate that melanoidins are comprised of a sugar-derived 'backbone' with supporting nitrogen subunits. This work shows that the relative concentrations of sugar and amino acid precursors are reflected in melanoidin compositions in much the same way that plant matter sources for humic substances show up in marine sediments. Stable carbon isotopic ratios for sugars and amino acids become 'imprinted' in melanoidins, whereas $\delta^{15}N$ ratios may indicate a fractionation characteristic of the melanoidin reaction. These data show that stable isotope ratios provide a powerful tool for evaluating the participation of the melanoidin reaction in the formation of humic substances in marine sediments.

It is interesting to note that humic and fulvic acids were isolated by Albert *et al.* (1988) from living and dead *Spartina alterniflora* plants of a Georgia salt marsh estuary. Stable carbon isotope data show -12 and -15% values for the fresh and dead plants, respectively.

Table 1.5. Isotopic data for selected melanoidins and humic substances. (Reproduced by permission from R. Ikan, T. Dorsey and I. R. Kaplan, *Anal. Chim. Acta*, **232**, 11, 1990. Copyright 1990, Elsevier Science Ltd)

Material	Expected		Determined	
	$\delta^{13}C$	$\delta^{13}N$	$\delta^{13}C$	$\delta^{13}N$
Melanoidin/humic substance				
Glu–Lys, 9:1	−11.50	+5.3	−12.56	+2.92
Gal–Iso, 9:1	−27.00	+5.2	−29.44	+6.10
Gal–Lys, 9:1	−26.80	+5.3	−26.16	+5.40
Gal–Lys, 1:1	−26.15	+5.3	−27.17	+4.16
Glu–Tyr 9:1	−11.56	+1.7	−17.40	−1.38
Glu–Lys, 1:1	−17.63	+5.3	−16.94	+4.78
Gal–Iso, 1:1	−27.11	+5.2	−27.18	+7.45
Glu–Tyr, 1:1	−18.11	+1.7	−19.30	−1.61
Glu–Tyr, 1:9	−24.66	+1.7	−19.20	+3.49
Marine humus (Gulf of Mexico)			−20.60	+4.00
Marine humus (Saanich inlet)			−21.20	+3.70
Walvis Bay (South Atlantic)			−18.46	+10.55
Izembek Lagoon (Alaska)			−18.43	+7.74
Tanner Basin (North Pacific)			−20.65	+9.10
Laguna Mormona (Baja Mexico)			−13.76	+1.70
Spartina alterniflora mud fulvics (Georgia salt marsh)			−18.33	
Terrestrial humus (Beaverhills soil)			−25.80	+4.70
Terrestrial humus (Washington peat)			−28.70	+5.70
Forest soil (Minnesota)			−26.67	+2.52
Peat (Staten Island, California)			−26.80	+2.70
Mangrove swamp (Australia)			−23.42	+4.31
Starting materials				
Glucose			−9.94	
Galactose			−26.96	
Isoleucine			−27.25	+5.20
Lysine			−25.33	+5.30
Tyrosine			−26.50	+1.68

THE FORMATION OF MELANOIDINS IN THE PRESENCE OF CLAYS

Only a few studies have been conducted to elucidate possible mechanisms of formation of melanoidin polymers in natural environments. Hedges (1978) had suggested that at higher pH values basic amino acids should condense more readily with sugars, thus increasing the rate of polymer formation. He also reported that the relative affinities of kaolinite and montmorillonite for dissolved melanoidins vary with pH, and montmorillonite removes more melanoidin than does kaolinite.

Taguchi and Sampei (1986) have synthesized melanoidins from glucose and glycine and glucose and alanine in the presence of clay minerals and calcium carbonate. Their experiments revealed that the 'melanoidins' consisted of a mixture of fulvic acid–humic acid and kerogen-like polymers. The kerogen-like polymers had elemental compositions similar to type II or type II/III kerogens. They also found that the rate of formation of melanoidins is highest in the presence of montmorillonite. This supports the hypothesis that kerogen-like melanoidins are formed by reacting only sugars and amino acids, which are present commonly in natural marine organisms with no kind of lignin-like starting material and having elemental compositions similar to type II/III kerogen with amorphous properties.

MODE OF FORMATION AND STRUCTURES OF NATURAL AND SYNTHETIC HUMIC SUBSTANCES

According to Bohn (1976), the mass of soil organic C (30.0×10^{14} kg) surpasses that of all other C reservoirs at the earth surface combined (atmospheric $CO_2 = 7 \times 10^{14}$ kg; biomass $C = 4.8 \times 10^{14}$ kg; fresh water $C = 2.5 \times 10^{14}$ kg; marine $C = 5-8 \times 10^{14}$ kg). Although 70–75% of the total soil C occurs in humic substances the structure and mode of formation of these complex natural products still remains a puzzle.

A wide variety of formation models have been suggested to explain the characteristics of humic substances found in different natural environments (Stevenson, 1982; Hedges, 1988). One of the two classes of models is the biopolymer degradation type, which assumes that polymerization occurs within cells via secondary metabolism to form biopolymers that are then partially degraded in the environment to produce humic substances. The other involves 'recombination' of the small organic molecules generated by the degradation of the original biopolymers (Figure 1.2). Hatcher and Spiker (1988) have assumed that the polymerized organic matter in sediments is produced by selective preservation of biopolymers.

BIOPOLYMER DEGRADATION MODELS

The biopolymer degradation model is based on the assumption that the humic polymers are assembled by living organisms via enzymatic mediation and that the resulting polymers should be refractory to microbial degradation. The most widely accepted biopolymer degradation model is the lignin–protein scheme proposed by Waksman (1932). It indicates a high degree of aromaticity of

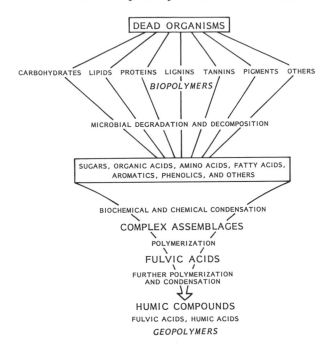

Figure 1.2. Formation of humic substances. (Reproduced by permission from M. A. Rashid, *Geochemistry of Marine Humic Substances*, Fig. 2.23, p. 59, 1985. Copyright 1985, Springer-Verlag, GmbH & Co. KG)

humic substances. A polysaccharide degradation model was suggested by Martin and Haider (1971).

ABIOTIC CONDENSATION MODELS

The abiotic condensation models are the most popular ones for the formation of marine and terrestrial humic substances. They account for the structural diversity of humic substances being formed from a complex mixture of precursors.

THE POLYPHENOL MODELS

This model is based on the assumption that a variety of phenolic compounds (except lignin) are the precursors of humic substances. A strong support in favour of the polyphenol model stems from the fact that the polymerization of quinones is an extremely facile reaction, especially at slightly basic pH or in the presence of nitrogenous substances as suggested by Stevenson (1982), and shown in Figure 1.3, which includes also the Maillard reaction pathway. The

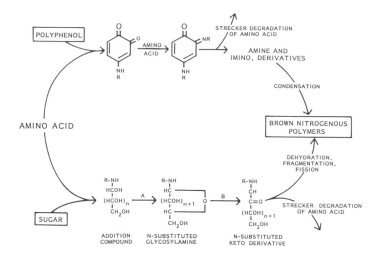

Figure 1.3. Suggested scheme for the formation of brown nitrogenous polymers in soils and sediments by condensation of amino acids with polyphenols (upper portion) and sugars through the Maillard reaction (lower portion). (Reproduced by permission from F. J. Stevenson, *Advances in Organic Geochemistry*, **39**, 1973, Fig. 1. Copyright 1973, Editions Technip)

proposed pathway was easily simulated in the laboratory with simple quinones, which rapidly condense with each other and with amino acids and ammonia, forming synthetic polymers that closely resemble those of soil humic substances (Ertel and Hedges, 1983; Mathur and Schnitzer, 1978). The polyphenol model has some drawbacks in explaining the formation of marine humic substances because phenols are not abundant in phytoplankton. Furthermore, the oxidation of phenols to quinones is difficult under the suboxic conditions existing beneath the surface of most coastal marine sediments. The high oxygen content (depending on the age of humic substances) leads to a C/O ratio of between 16 in recently formed humic substances from waters and 25 in the oldest humic acids (lignites), which cannot be accounted for by structural proposals, most of which were based on aromatic benzenoid structures. Thus, Fuchs (1931), Kononova (1966) and Flaig (1960) have proposed various structures of humic acids. Schnitzer and Khan (1972) concluded that fulvic acids consist in part of phenolic and benzenecarboxylic acids held together through hydrogen bonds to form a polymeric structure of considerable stability. Buffle's (1977) model suggests a structure of fulvic acid. A hypothetical structure of humic acid showing free and bound phenolic hydroxyl groups, quinone structures, oxygen as bridge units and carbonyl on aromatic rings was proposed by Stevenson (1982). Based on the Waksman's lignin model, many researchers suggested that humic

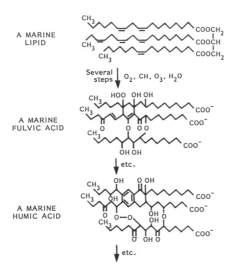

Figure 1.4. Representative structures in the dynamic continuum of fulvic and humic acid formation. For more details see Harvey *et al.* (1983). (Reprinted with permission from G. R. Harvey, D. A. Boran, L. A. Chesal and J. M. Tokar, *Marine Chemistry*, **12**, 119, 1983. Copyright 1983, Elsevier Science)

substances have a high degree of aromaticity. In more recent studies, several authors have found a relatively high proportion of aliphatic chains in aqueous humic substances (Wilson *et al.*, 1978; De Haan *et al.*, 1979). These findings are in significant contrast to soil humic substances. The structural units of fulvic and humic acids published by Liao *et al.* (1982) are similar to those proposed by Bergmann (1978), who studied humic substances of activated sludge systems. Bergmann's proposed humic units also contain relatively small amounts of aromatic rings, with the aliphatic polyethers being the dominant building blocks.

Martin and Pierce (1975) proposed an oxidative polymerization pathway of phenolic derivatives involving amino sugar units. A polyunsaturated lipid model was suggested by Harvey *et al.* (1983) (Figure 1.4). It involves autooxidative crosslinking reactions between adjacent polyunsaturated fatty acids (found in many types of marine phytoplankton) which are exposed to sunlight at the ocean surface. Harvey's mechanism explains the presence of relatively aliphatic, oxygen-rich humic substances in sea water. It was supported by laboratory-simulated experiments with polyunsaturated fats which produced humic-type condensation products which resembled dissolved humic substances isolated from sea water (Harvey and Boran, 1985). Despite the appealing characteristics of this model, the polyunsaturated lipid model has some problems. Thus, the stable carbon isotopic compositions that have been

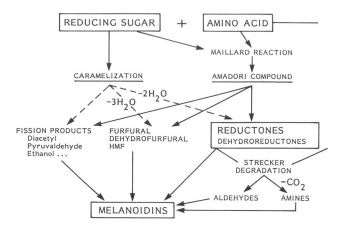

Figure 1.5. The Maillard reaction

reported for total dissolved organic carbon (DOC) of HS isolated from sea water more closely resembled those measured in the nonlipid components of local marine plankton (Stuermer and Harvey, 1974; Meyers-Schulte and Hedges, 1986). Furthermore, the proposed model does not include a clear mechanism for the incorporation of nitrogen into the lipid-derived photolysis products (Harvey and Boran, 1985).

The melanoidin or 'browning reaction' model which involves condensation reactions between simple sugars and amino acids was first introduced by Maillard (1913) (Figure 1.5) and has been periodically studied ever since (e.g. Hoering, 1973; Nissenbaum and Kaplan, 1972; Hedges, 1978; Ikan *et al.*, 1986b).

The melanoidin model is especially favorable for marine environments where the two precursors, sugars and amino acids, are among the most abundant constituents of all living organisms and will combine under reducing as well as oxidizing conditions. It was found that the condensation of reducing sugars with basic amino acids is kinetically favored over reactions with other amino acid types, leading to nitrogen-rich polymers that resemble marine humic substances in many of their chemical and spectroscopic properties. Rubinsztain *et al.* (1984) have proposed possible pathways of melanoidin formation (Figure 1.6).

Ikan *et al.* (1986a) have suggested that the melanoidin reaction plays a significant role in the process of formation of the core of humic substances in nature. The ^{13}C-CP-MAS NMR studies indicated the presence of significant absorptions in the aromatic region which probably correspond to furanoid and furfural-like structures, to the substituted hydroxyalkylcyclopentenone (sugar origin) and/or hydroxy alkyl furanone as well as certain pyrrole moieties. The

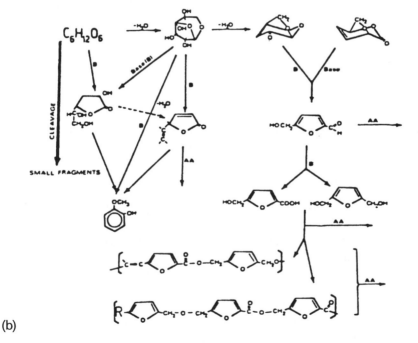

(a)

(b)

Figure 1.6. (a) Amino acids (AA)–SG condensation and structural units in polymerization of melanoidins: nitrogen-containing moieties. (b) Sugar (SG) moiety-based proposed pathways for melanoidin polymerization 'backbone' structure. (Reprinted with permission from Y. Rubinsztain, P. Ioselis, R. Ikan and Z. Aizenshtat, *Organic Geochemistry*, **6**, 804, 1984. Copyright 1984, Elsevier Science Ltd)

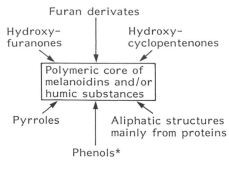

Figure 1.7. Proposed nonbenzenoid polymeric core of humic substances. (Reproduced by permission from R. Ikan, P. Ioselis, Y. Rubinsztain, Z. Aizenshtat, R. Pugmire, L. Anderson and R. Ishiwatari, *Naturwissenschaften*, **73**, 150, 1986. Copyright 1986, Springer-Verlag GmbH & Co. KG)

proposed nonbezenoid polymeric core of humic substances is presented in Figure 1.7.

Cowie *et al.* (1992) showed that sugars and amino acids which reach the sediment surface go through a diagenetic change to form refractory compounds. Recently, Mayer (1994) has shown that sedimentary organic matter in soil exists in thin films, mostly covering very small pores (< 8 nm), which protects them against bacterial grazing.

Thus, while the pathway of formation of geopolymers is unresolved, there is evidence that the Maillard reaction may be an important driving force in the accumulation of resistant, high molecular weight, organic matter in sediments. It is probable that the two models or pathways complement each other. For example, melanoidin can absorb a very wide range of hydrophobic and hydrophilic substances. They can also form a three-dimensional, porous structure which can host a wide variety of guest compounds, either by mechanical trapping or through some sort of weak bonding such as hydrogen bonds. The algal-derived biopolymers and the melanoidins can thus coexist in soils and sediments.

Recently, Kato and Tsuchida (1981) have proposed the structure shown in Figure 1.8 as a more favorable structure for melanoidins, rather than one based on the phenolic group. Wershaw (1986) has developed a generalized model of the physical–chemical state of humic substances which is consistent with their

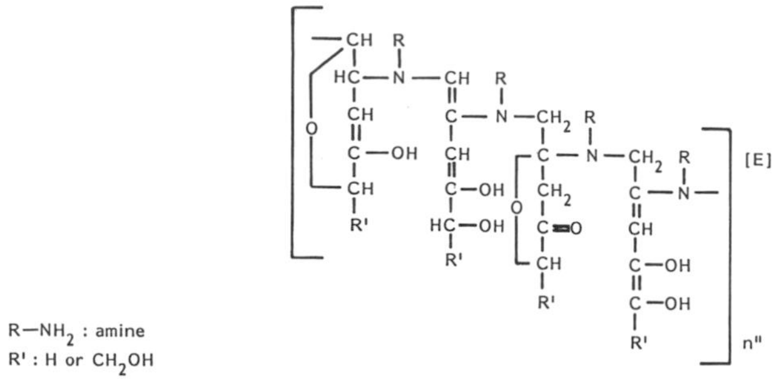

R—NH$_2$: amine
R' : H or CH$_2$OH

Figure 1.8. Possible repeating units of polymeric brown products and their precursors

observed properties. In this model it is proposed that the humics in soil and sediments consist of a number of different oligomers and simple compounds which result from the partial degradation of plant remains. These degradation products are stabilized by incorporation into humic aggregates bound together by weak bonding, such as hydrogen bonding, pi bonding and hydrophobic interactions. The resulting structures are similar to micelles or membranes, in which the interiors of the structures are hydrophobic and the exteriors are hydrophilic. This model provides a means of understanding the movement and bonding of hydrophobic organic pollutants in soils and sediments. It also provides a model for metal interactions in these polymeric substances.

In connection with the 'aliphatic versus aromatic structure' controversy of humic substances, it should be pointed out that it was never completely understood how humic substances made up predominantly of aromatic structural elements could be converted into the aliphatics found almost exclusively in petroleum under the relatively mild conditions associated with its formation. Since the aliphatic structural units present in humic substances cannot further be degraded microbiologically, they could form the basis for aliphatic geopolymers and petroleum. It has been recently suggested by Bayer and Kutubuddin (1981) that petroleum is predominantly formed from lignin-free aquatic biomass and coal, of vegetable origin.

Recent works by Taguchi and Sampei (1986) on synthetic melanoidins have pointed out that the plot on the Van Krevelen diagram showing the hydrogen and carbon composition to be acid soluble (fulvic acid-like) and acid insoluble (humic acid-like) are in the same region as types II and III kerogens.

It has been suggested that the structural features of melanoidins might be similar to the chemical models drawn by Behar and Vandenbroucke (1987) for humic substances. The current rapid developments of new analytical methods (Ikan and Crammer, 1982) might soon furnish more information for the most complex structures of humic substances.

MELANOIDINS AS MATRICES FOR PREBIOTIC ACTIVITY

Nissenbaum *et al.* (1975) have suggested the involvement of melanoidin polymers in prebiotic activity. The following is based on this speculative article.

MELANOIDIN AND THE PREBIOTIC SOUP

A basic feature of most theories of chemical evolution is the assumption that abiogenic production of organic monomers led to the accumulation of simple molecules in the primitive water bodies, which could have been either oceanic or lacustrine. The resulting organic-rich solution has been given various names such as 'nutrient broth' or 'prebiotic soup'.

Contrary to the earlier suggestion that essentially all stages of chemical evolution occurred in the sea, it is now generally accepted that the concentration of the 'soup' was probably too small for efficient synthesis of biopolymers (Miller and Orgel, 1974). Other suggestions (Matthews, 1974) envisaged the land surface of the earth to be covered by proteinaceous material and other products of atmospheric photochemistry. Even this terrestrial model assumes that at some stage the polymers were washed into the oceans where the evolution of enzyme reaction chains occurred. It is reasonable to assume that concomitant with the production of simple organic molecules and their accumulation in the ocean, there would have been an opposing mechanism of condensation of the accumulating amino acids (or amines) and carbohydrates to form the insoluble polymers of the melanoidin type. Hence, an 'organic-rich soup' had to be continually forming to provide precursors for nucleic acids and enzyme synthesis.

THE POSSIBLE ROLE OF MELANOIDINS AS PROTOENZYMATIC EXTERNAL ELECTRON ACCEPTORS

Considering the presumed anoxic nature of the prebiotic environment, it is very frequently assumed that most primitive metabolic systems were capable of obtaining energy through reactions in which organic matter, rather than oxygen, acted as the terminal electron acceptors. Most of the coenzymes utilized in anaerobic oxidation–reduction processes contain heterocyclic nitrogen bases as part of their structure, such as nicotinamides and flavins.

It has been suggested that under prebiotic conditions, melanoidins may have acted as primitive coenzymes, because they contain large amounts of heterocyclic nitrogen, suggesting their similarity to some of the oxidation–reduction coenzymes. The melanoidins also contain appreciable concentrations of long-lived free radicals, probably due to a semi-quinone structure, possibly equivalent to flavine coenzymes. Thus melanoidins may have had a role in some primitive oxidation–reduction systems. The flavine coenzymes contain base and transition metals which take part in the oxidation–reduction chain. These metals are Zn, Mo, Cu and Fe. These metals are also concentrated in marine humic substances (Harvey and Boran, 1985). Because melanoidins and some of the coenzymes have many properties in common, it has been suggested that melanoidins may have acted as primeval, external electron acceptors in prebiotic times. It is also possible that melanoidins may have acted as an adsorptive matrix for both micro- and macromolecules, such as amino acid and proteins.

Nissenbaum and Serban (1987) have shown that marine sediments, down to 270 m below the sediment–water interface, retain some peroxidase activity. This was interpreted to be a result of a humic substance–enzyme complex which is stable toward degradation. Similarly, stable complexes were made synthetically (Serban and Nissenbaum, 1986) and the complexes were much more resistant to heat and enzymatic degradation than the free enzymes. Thus, geopolymers cannot only act as primeval enzymes, but have the ability to absorb and stabilize externally formed enzymes.

REFERENCES

Abelson, P. H., and Hare, P. E. (1971). Reactions of amino acids with natural and artificial humics and kerogens, *Carnegie Inst. Washington Yearbook*, **69**, 327–34.

Aizenshtat, Z., Rubinsztain, Y., Ioselis, P., Miloslavsky, I., and Ikan, R. (1987). Long-lived free radicals study of stepwise pyrolyzed melanoidins and humic substances, *Org. Geochem.*, **11**, 65–71.

Albert, J. J., Zdenek, F., Price, M. T., Williams, D. J., and Williams, M. C. (1988). Elemental composition, stable carbon isotope ratios and spectrophotometric properties of humic substances occurring in a salt marsh estuary, *Org. Geochem.*, **12**, 455–67.

Andrew, E. R. (1972). The narrowing of NMR spectra of solids by high speed specimen rotation and the resolution of chemical shift and spin multiplet structures of solids. In J. W. Ensley, J. Feehez and L. H. Satcliffe (eds.), *Progress in NMR Spectroscopy*, Vol. 8, Part I. Pergamon Press, New York, pp. 1–39.

Bayer E., and Kutubuddin, M. (1981). Oil from detritus and waste, *Bild der Wissenschaft*, **18**(9), 68–77.

Behar, F., and Vandenbroucke, M. (1987). Chemical modeling of kerogens, *Org. Geochem.*, **1**, 15–24.

Benzing-Purdie, L., Ripmeester, J. A., and Ratcliffe, C. I. (1985). Effect of temperature on Maillard reaction products, *J. Agric. Food Chem.*, **33**, 31–3.

Bergmann, W. (1978). PhD. Thesis, Tubingen University.

Bohn, H. L. (1976). Estimate of organic carbon in world soils, *Soil Sci. Soil Am. J.*, **40**, 468–70.

Borkovsky, O. K. (1965). Sources of organic matter in marine basins, *Mar. Geol.*, **3**, 5–31.

Buffle, J. (1977). Les substances humique et leur interaitions avec les ions mineraux, Conference Proc. de la Commission d'Hydrologie Appliquee de l'A.G.H.T.M., l'Universite Orsay, pp. 3–10.

Chuang, I. S., Maciel, G., and Myers, G. (1984). ^{13}C NMR study of curing in furfuryl alcohol resins, *Macromolecules*, **17**, 1087–90.

Cowie, G. L., Hedges, J. I., and Calvert, S. E. (1992). Sources and relative reactivities of amino acids, neutral sugars and lignin in an intermittently anoxic fjord, *Geochim. Costmochim. Acta*, **56**, 1963–78.

De Haan, H., De Boer, T., and Halma, G. (1979). Curie point pyrolysis/mass spectrometry of fulvic acids from Tjeukmeer, The Netherlands, *Freshwater Biol.*, **9**, 315–17.

Dereppe, J. M., Moreaux, C., and Debyser, Y. (1980). Investigation of marine and terrestrial humic substances of ^{1}H and ^{13}C nuclear magnetic resonance and infrared spectroscopy, *Org. Geochem.*, **2**, 117–124.

Durand, B., Nicaise, G., Roucache, M., Van Denbroucke, M., and Hagemann, M. W. (1977). Etude geochimique d'une serie de charbons. In R. Campos and J. Goni (eds.), *Advances in Organic Geochemistry*, 1983, Pergamon Press, Oxford, pp. 601–31.

Enders, C., and Theis, K. (1938). Die melanoidine und ihre Beziehung zu den Huminsaure, *Brennst. Chem.*, **19**, 402–7.

Engel, M. H., Rafalska-Bloch, J., Schielbein, C. F., Zemberge, J. E., and Serban, H. (1986). Simulated diagenesis and catagenesis of marine kerogen precursors. Melanoidin as model systems for light hydrocarbons generation, *Org. Geochem.*, **10**, 1073–9.

Ertel, J. R., and Hedges, J. I. (1983). Bulk chemical and spectroscopic properties of marine and terrestrial humic acids, melanoidins and catechol-based synthetic polymers. In R. F. Christman, and E. T. Gjessing (eds.), *Aquatic and Terrestrial Humic Materials*, Ann Arbor Science, Michigan, pp. 143–63.

Flaig, W. (1960). Comparative chemical investigations on natural humic compounds and their model substances, *Sci. Proc. Roy. Dublin Soc.*, **4**, 49–62.

Flaig, W. (1964). Effects of micro-organisms in the transformation of lignin to humic substances, *Geochim. Cosmochim. Acta*, **28**, 1523–35.

Fuchs, W. (1931). *Die Chemie der Kohle,*, Springer-Verlag, Berlin.

Gillam, A. H., and Wilson, M. A. (1985). Pyrolysis–GC–MS and NMR studies of dissolved sea water humic substances and isolates of a marine diatom, *Org. Geochem.*, **8**, 15–25.

Gonzalez Vila, F. J., Lentz, H., and Ludeman, J. D. (1976). FT ^{13}C nuclear magnetic resonance spectra of natural humic substances, *Biochem. Biophys. Res. Commun.*, **72**, 1065–9.

Gonzalez Vila, F. J., Ludeman, J. D., and Martin, F. (1983). ^{13}C NMR structural features of soil humic acids and their methylated hydrolyzed and extracted derivatives, *Geoderma*, **31**, 3–15.

Harvey, G. T., and Boran, P. A. (1985). Geochemistry of humic substances in sea water. In G. R. Aiken, D. M. McKnight, R. L. Wershaw and P. MacCarthy (eds.) *Humic Substances in Soil, Sediment and Water*, John Wiley & Sons, New York, pp. 147–80.

Harvcy, G. R., Boran, D. A., Chesal, L. A., and Tokar, J. M. (1983). The structure of marine fulvic and humic acids, *Mar. Chem.*, **12**, 199–232.

Hatcher P. G., and Spiker, E. C. (1988). Selective degradation of plant biomolecules. In F. H. Frimmel and R. F. Christman (eds.), *Humic Substances and Their Role in the Environment*, John Wiley & Sons, New York.

Hatcher, P. G., Rowan, R., and Mattingly, M. (1980a). ^{1}H and ^{13}C NMR of marine humic acids, *Org. Geochem.*, **2**, 77–85.

Hatcher, P. G., Van der Hart, D. L., and Earl, W. L. (1980b). Use of solid-state ^{13}C NMR in structural studies of humic acids and humin from Holoane sediments, *Org. Geochem.*, **2**, 87–92.

Hatcher, P. G., Maciel, G. E., and Dennis, L. W. (1981). Aliphatic structure of humic acids, a clue to their origin, *Org. Geochem.*, **3**, 43–8.

Hayase, F., and Kato, H. (1981). Volatile compounds formed by thermal degradation of non-dialyzable melanoidins prepared from a sugar-amino acid reaction system, *Agric. Biol. Chem.*, **45**, 2559–69.

Hedges, J. L. (1978). The formation and clay mineral reaction of melanoidins, *Geochim. Cosmochim. Acta*, **42**, 69–76.

Hedges, J. L. (1988). Polymerization of humic substances in natural environments. In P. H. Frimmel and R. F. Christman (eds.), *Humic Substances and Their Role in the Environment*, John Wiley & Sons, New York, pp. 45–58.

Hedges, J. L., and Parker, P. L. (1976). Land-derived organic matter in surface sediments from the Gulf of Mexico, *Geochim. Cosmochim. Acta*, **40**, 1019–29.

Hicks, K. B., and Feather, M. S. (1975). Studies on the mechanism of formation of 4-hydroxy-5-methyl-3(2*H*)-furanone component of beef flavor from Amadori products, *J. Agric. Food Chem.*, **23**, 957–60.

Hodge, J. E. (1953). Chemistry of browning reaction in model system, *Agric. Food Chem.*, **1**, 926–43.

Hoering, R. C. (1973). A comparison of melanoidins and humic acid, *Carnegie Inst. Washington Yearbook*, **72**, 682–90.

Ikan, R., and Crammer, B. (1992). *Organic Chemistry: Compound Detection. Encyclopedia of Physical Science and Technology*, Vol. 12, Academic Press, New York, pp. 46–81.

Ikan, R., Ioselis, P., Rubinsztain, Y., Aizenshtat, Z., Pugmire, R., Anderson, L. L., and Ishiwatari, R. (1986a). Carbohydrate origin of humic substances, *Naturwissen.*, **73**, 150–1.

Ikan, R., Rubinsztain, Y., Ioselis, P., Aizenshtat, Z., Pugmire, P., Anderson, L. L., and Woolfenden, W. R. (1986b). Carbon-13 cross polarized magic angle samples spinning nuclear magnetic resonance of melanoidins, *Org. Geochem.*, **9**, 199–212.

Ikan, R., Dorsey, T., and Kaplan, I. R. (1990). Characterization of natural and synthetic humic substances (melanoidins) by stable carbon and nitrogen isotope measurements and elemental analysis, *Anal. Chim. Acta*, **232**, 11–18.

Ishiwatari, R., Marinaga, S., Yamamoto, S., Michihara, T., Rubinsztain, Y., Ioselis, P., Aizenshtat, Z., and Ikan, R. (1986). Characterization of synthetic humic substances (melanoidins) by alkaline permanganate oxidation, *Org. Geochem.*, **9**, 11–25.

Kato, H., and Tsuchida, H. (1981). Formation of melanoidin structure by pyrolysis and oxidation, *Prog. Food Nutr. Sci.*, **5**, 147–56.

Kononova, M. M. (1966). *Soil Organic Matter*, Pergamon Press, Oxford, 544 pp.

Lessig, V., and Bates, W. (1982). Modell-untersuchungen zur Maillard Reaction VII: Freie radicale in einigen ausgesuchten melanoidinen, *Z. Leben Unters. Forsch.*, **175**, 13–14.

Liao, W., Christman, R. F., Johnson, J. D., and Millington, D. S. (1982). Structural characterization of aquatic humic material, *Environ. Sci. Technol.*, **6**, 403–10.

Machihara, T., and Ishiwatari, R. (1983). Evaluation of alkaline permanganate oxidation method for the characterization of young kerogen, *Org. Geochem.*, **5**, 111–19.

Maillard, L. C. (1913). Formation des matieres humiques par action de polypeptides sur sucre, *Comp. Rend. Acad. Sci.*, **156**, 148–9.

Martin, J. P., and Haider, K. (1971). Microbial activity in solution in relation to soil humus formation, *Soil Sci.*, **111**, 54–63.

Martin, D. F., and Pierce, P. A. (1975). A convenient method of analysis of humic acids in freshwater, *Environ. Lett.*, **1**, 49–52.

Martin, F., Saiz-Jimenez, C., and Gonzalez-Vila, F. J. (1981). The persulfate oxidation of soil humic acid, *Soil Sci.*, **132**, 200–3.

Mathur, S. P., and Schnitzer, M. (1978). A chemical and spectroscopic characterization of some synthetic analogues of humic acids, *Soil Sci. Soc. Am. J.*, **42**, 591–5.

Matthews, C. N. (1974). The origin of proteins: heteropolypeptides from hydrogen cyanide and water. In J. Oro, S. L. Miller, C. Ponnamperuma and R. S. Young (eds.), *Cosmochemical Evolution and the Origins of Life*, pp. 155–62.

Mauron, J. (1981) Maillard reaction in food: a critical review from the nutritional standpoint, *Prog. Food Nutr. Sci.*, **5**, 5–35.

Mayer, L. M. (1994). Relationships between mineral surfaces and organic carbon concentrations in soils and sediments, *Chem. Geol.*, **114**, 347–83.

Meyers-Schulte, K. J., and Hedges, J. I. (1986). Molecular evidence for a terrestrial component of organic matter dissolved in ocean water, *Nature*, **321**, 61–3.

Mikita, M. A., Steelink, C., and Wershaw, R. L. (1981). Carbon-13 enriched nuclear magnetic resonance method for the determination of hydroxyl functionality in humic substances, *Anal. Chem.*, **53**, 1715–17.

Miller, S. L., and Orgel, L. E. (1974). *The Origins of Life on Earth*, Prentice-Hall, Englewood Cliffs, New Jersey.

Nissenbaum, A. (1973). The organic geochemistry of marine and terrestrial humic substances, *Adv. Org. Geochem.*, **39**, 52.

Nissenbaum, A., and Kaplan, J. R. (1972). Chemical and isotopic evidence for the *in situ* origin of marine humic substances, *Limnol. Oceanogr.*, **17**, 570–82.

Nissenbaum, A., and Serban, A. (1987). Enzymatic activity associated with humic substances in deep sediments from the Cariaco trench and Walvis ridge, *Geochim. Cosmochim. Acta*, **51**, 371–8.

Nissenbaum, A., Kenyon, D. H., and Oro, J. (1975). On the possible role or organic melanoidin polymers as matrices for prebiotic activity, *J. Mol. Evol.*, **6**, 253–70.

Ogner, G. (1973). Permanganate oxidation of methylated and unmethylated fulvic acid, humic acid and humin isolated from raw humus, *Acta Chem. Scand.*, **27**, 1601–2.

Ogner, G. (1979). The ^{13}C nuclear magnetic resonance spectrum of methylated humic acid, *Soil. Biol. Biochem.*, **11**, 105–8.

Olsson, K., Pernemalm, P. A. and Theander, O. (1981). Reaction products and mechanism in some simple model systems, *Prog. Food Nutr. Sci.*, **5**, 47–55.

Preston, C. M., and Schnitzer, M. (1984). Effects of chemical modifications and extractants on the carbon-13 NMR spectra of humic materials, *Soil Sci. Am. J.*, **48**, 305–11.

Pugmire, R. J., Zilm, K. W., Woolfenden, W. R., Grant, D. M., Dyrkacz, G. R., Bloomquist, C. A. A., and Horwitz, E. P. (1982). Carbon-13 NMR spectra of macerals separated from individual coals, *Org. Geochem.*, **4**, 79–84.

Riffaldi, R., and Schnitzer, M. (1972). Effects of diverse experimental conditions on ESR spectra of humic substances, *Geoderma*, **8**, 1–10.

Rubinsztain, Y., Ioselis, P., Ikan, R., and Aizenshtat, Z. (1984). Investigations on the structural units of melanoidins, *Org. Geochem.*, **6**, 791–804.

Schnitzer, M. (1977). Recent findings on the characterization of humic substances extracted from soil from widely differing climatic zones. In *Soil Organic Matter Studies*, Vol. 2, International Atomic Energy Agency, pp. 117–32.

Schnitzer, M., and de Serra, M. I. (1973). The chemical degradation of humic acid, *Can. J. Chem.*, **51**, 1554–66.

Schnitzer, M., and Khan, S. U. (1972). *Humic Substances in the Environment*, Marcel Dekker, New York.

Senesi, N., and Schnitzer, M. (1977). Effects of pH, reaction time, chemical reduction and irradiation on ESR spectra of fulvic acid, *Soil Sci.*, **123**, 224–34.

Serban, A., and Nissenbaum, A. (1986). Humic acid association with peroxidase and catalase, *Soil Biol. Biotech.*, **18**, 41–4.

Shaw, P. E., Tatum, J. H., and Berry, R. E. (1968). Base-catalyzed fructose degradation and its relation to non-enzymatic browning, *J. Agric. Food Chem.*, **16**, 979–82.

Steelink, C. (1964). Free radical studies of lignin degradation products and soil humic acids, *Geochim. Cosmochim. Acta*, **28**, 1615–22.

Stevenson, F. J. (1973). Nonbiological transformations of amino acids in soils and sediments, *Adv. Org. Geochem.*, 701–14.

Stevenson, F. J. (1982). *Humus Chemistry: Genesis, Compositions, Reactions*, John Wiley & Sons, New York.

Stuermer, D. H., and Harvey, G. R. (1974). Humic substances from sea water, *Nature*, **250**, 480–1.

Taguchi, K., and Sampei, Y. (1986). The formation and clay mineral and $CaCo_3$ association reactions of melanoidins, *Org. Geochem.*, **10**, 1081–9.

Tissot, B., Durand, B., Espitalie, J., and Combaz, A. (1974). Influence of nature and diagenesis of organic matter in formation of petroleum, *Am. Assoc. Petrol. Geol. Bull.*, **58**, 499–506.

Waksman, S. A. (1932). *Humus*, Williams and Wilkins, Baltimore, Maryland.

Wershaw, R. L. (1986). A new method for humic materials and their interactions with hydrophobic organic chemicals in soil–water or sediment–water systems, *J. Contaminant Hydrology*, **1**, 29–45.

Wilson, M. A., and Goh, K. M. (1977). Proton-decoupled pulse Fourier-transform ^{13}C magnetic resonance of soil organic matter, *J. Soil Sci.*, **32**, 167–86.

Wilson, M. A., Jones, A. J., and Williamson, B. (1978). Nuclear magnetic resonance spectrosocpy of humic materials, *Nature*, **276**, 487–9.

Wilson, M. A., Pugmire, R. J., Zilm, K. W., Goh, K. M., Heng, S., and Grant, D. M. (1981). Cross-polarization ^{13}C-NMR spectroscopy with 'magic angle' spinning characterizes organic matter in whole soils, *Nature*, **294**, 648–50.

Wolfrom, M. L., Cavalieri, L. F., and Cavalieri, D. K. (1947). Chemical interaction of amino compounds and sugars. II. Methylation experiments, *J. Am. Chem. Soc.*, **69**, 2411–13.

2

Thermal Generation of Maillard Aromas

CHI-TANG HO

Department of Food Science, Cook College, New Jersey Agricultural Experiment
Station, Rutgers State University, New Brunswick, New Jersey

INTRODUCTION

One of the major reactions involved in the formation of food aromas during
thermal processing is the Maillard reaction or nonenzymatic browning
reaction. The subject of the Maillard reaction has been extensively reviewed
in many books and articles.[1-6] The wide variety of aromas generated in the
Maillard reaction results from the large number of reactants that can combine
during the thermal reaction.[7]

A summary of the Maillard reaction is given in Scheme 1.[8] The first step
involves Schiff base formation between the carbonyl group of a reducing sugar
and the free amino group of an amino acid, peptide or protein. These Schiff
bases can rearrange to form reactive intermediates such as 1-deoxyglycosones
or 3-deoxyglycosones through amino–deoxyaldose or ketose by Amadori or
Heyns rearrangements. Structures of these two important intermediates are
shown in Figure 2.1. These 1-deoxyglycosones or 3-deoxyglycosones can
undergo a retro-aldolization reaction to produce reactive α-dicarbonyl
compounds, such as pyruvaldehyde and diacetyl. It is these reactive
compounds that will interact with other components such as ammonia and
hydrogen sulfide to produce many significant flavor compounds.

Many aroma compounds derived from the Maillard reaction are odor-active
components of processed foods. Table 2.1 lists potent odorants formed by the
Maillard reaction as detected by aroma extract dilution analysis.

The Maillard Reaction: Consequences for the Chemical and Life Sciences. Edited by Raphael Ikan
©1996 John Wiley & Sons Ltd

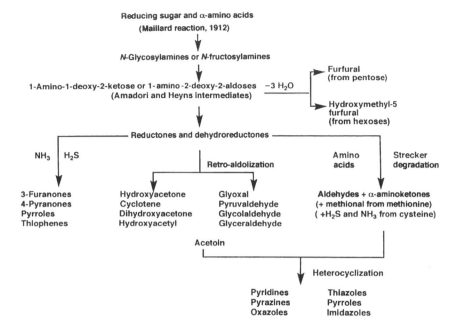

Scheme 1. Formation of Maillard aroma compounds in food products. (Reproduced from Ref. 8 by permission of Ellis Horwood Publishers)

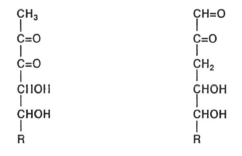

1-Deoxyosone   **3-Deoxyosone**

Figure 2.1. Structures of 1-deoxyglycosone and 3-deoxyglycosone

Table 2.1. Potent odorants formed by the Maillard reaction

Compound	Detected by AEDA[a] in foods[b]							Identified in model system
	RC	WBC	RBC	SM	RM	RS	P	
3-Methylbutanal	+	+	+					
2,3-Butanedione	+	+	+	+	+			
2,3-Pentanedione	+				+			
Methional	+	+	+	+	+			
Phenylacetaldehyde	+	+	+	+				
2-Furfurylthiol	+			+		+	+	
2-Acetyl-1-pyrroline			+		+		+	+
2-Propionyl-1-pyrroline							+	
2-Acetyltetrahydropyridine			+				+	+
2-Acetyl-2-thiazoline				+	+			
2-Ethyl-3,5-dimethyl-pyrazine	+	+	+	+	+	+	+	
2,3-Diethyl-5-methyl-pyrazine	+			+	+	+	+	
2,5-Dimethyl-4-hydroxy-3(2H)-furanone	+	+	+	+	+	+		
4,5-Dimethyl-3-hydroxy-2(5H)-furanone	+		+	+	+			
5-Ethyl-3-hydroxy-4-methyl-2(5H)-furanone	+		+		+			

[a]AEDA: aroma extract dilution analysis.
[b]RC: roasted coffee;[9] WBC: wheat bread crust;[10] RBC: rye bread crust;[11] SM: stewed meat;[12] RM: roasted meat;[13] RS: roasted sesame;[14] P: popcorn.[15]

FORMATION OF AMINO COMPOUND-SPECIFIC MAILLARD REACTION AROMAS

CYSTEINE-SPECIFIC COMPOUNDS

Thermal degradation of nonsulfur-containing amino acids leads to the formation of the corresponding amines via decarboxylation. Thermal degradation of sulfur-containing amino acids such as cysteine produces additional reactive breakdown products. Many potential possibilities exist for these products to interact and form various types of heterocyclic compounds which usually contribute considerably to the characteristic food flavors. Therefore, sulfur-containing amino acids are generally recognized as very important precursors of food flavors.

Boelens *et al.*[16] studied the degradation of cysteine/cystine in terms of primary and secondary products. They postulated a mechanism for the interaction between acetaldehyde and hydrogen sulfide (Figure 2.2). The

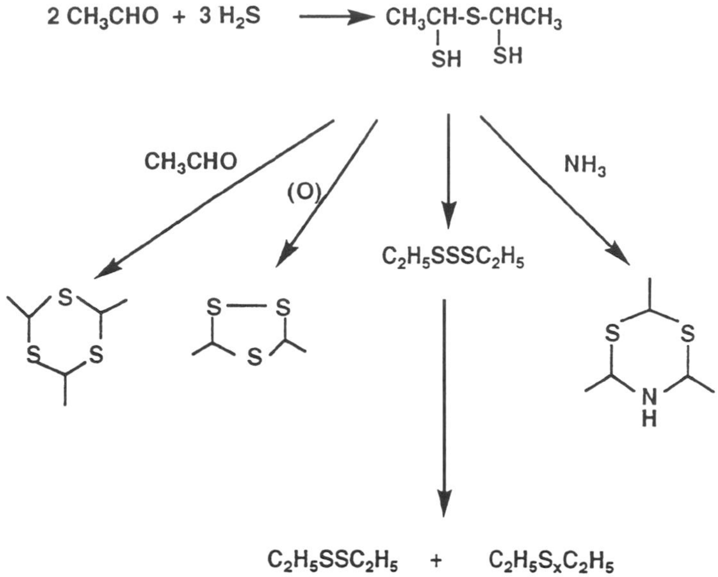

Figure 2.2. Mechanism of the interaction between acetaldehyde and hydrogen sulfide. (Adapted and reprinted with permission from Ref. 16. Copyright 1974, American Chemical Society)

interaction of acetaldehyde and hydrogen sulfide forms bis(1-mercaptoethyl) sulfide, which oxidized to 3,5-dimethyl-1,2,4-trithiolane in the presence of acid or to 2,4,6-trimethylperhydro-1,3,5-dithiazine in the presence of ammonia. In addition, bis(1-mercaptoethyl) sulfide can be disproportionationed into different sulfides including ethyl disulfide and ethyl trisulfide.

Shu *et al.*[17,18] studied the pH effect on the thermal degradation of cysteine in dilute aqueous solution. A vigorous degradation was observed at pH 5.1 which is the isoelectric point of cysteine. At pH 2.2, the major components were 1,2,3-trithia-5-cycloheptene and 2-thiophenethiol. The 1,2,3-trithia-5-cycloheptene was judged to resemble roasted onion and roasted meat odor. Figure 2.3 shows the formation of 1,2,3-trithia-5-cycloheptene by the condensation of mercaptoacetaldehyde and acetaldehyde.

Tressl *et al.*[19] characterized cysteine-specific products using cysteine–xylose, cysteine–glucose and cysteine–rhamnose model systems. Thirty cysteine-specific compounds were identified, some of which are listed in Table 2.2. Many of these compounds have been characterized as impact compounds in food flavors. Furfuryl mercaptan identified in the cysteine–pentose system has been known as an impact component of roasted coffee[20] and 2-methyl-3-mercaptothiophene is an important flavor compound in roasted/cooked beef.[21]

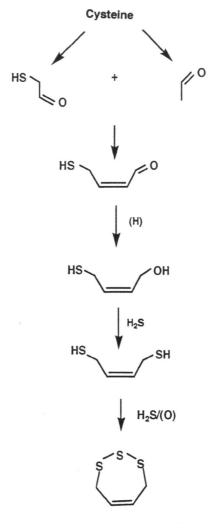

Figure 2.3. Mechanism for the formation of 1,2,3-trithia-5-cycloheptene. (Reprinted with permission from Ref. 18. Copyright 1985, American Chemical Society)

Table 2.3 showed the quantitative comparison of volatile compounds formed in six model systems containing either cysteine or cysteine-containing tripeptide, glutathione (γ-Glu–Cys–Gly).[22-24] The degradation of cysteine alone produced the greatest amount of volatile compounds compared with the interaction of either glucose or 2,4-decadienal. Glutathione was less reactive than cysteine in the reaction with carbonyl compounds. The quantitation also shows that, in the presence of carbonyls, the formation of thiophene was

Table 2.2. Some cysteine-specific Maillard products

From Strecker degradation
    Mercaptoacetaldehyde
    3,5-Dimethyl-1,2,4-trithiolane
    2,4,6-Trimethylperhydro-1,3,5-dithiazine
    3,6-Dimethyl-1,2,4,5-tetrathiane
    1,2,3-Trithia-5-cycloheptene
    2-Methyl-1,3-dithiolane
    3-Methyl-1,2-dithiolan-4-one

From cysteine–pentose model system
    2-Mercaptopropionic acid
    2-Methyl-3-mercaptothiophene
    2-Hydroxymethyl-4-thiolanone
    2-Methyl-4-thianone
    4-Hydroxy-5-methyl-3($2H$)-thiophenone
    2-Methyl-3($2H$)-thiophenone
    2-Methyl-3-thiolanone
    2-Methyl-4,5-dihydrothiophene
    Furfuryl mercaptan

From cysteine–hexose model system
    4-Hydroxy-2,4-dimethyl-3($2H$)-thiophenone
    2,4-Dihydroxy-2,5-dimethyl-3($2H$)-thiophenone
    2-Hydroxy-2,5-dimethyl-3($2H$)-thiophenone
    2,5-Dimethyl-3-thiolanone

Table 2.3. Quantitation of classified compounds in different model systems[a] (mg/mole)

Compound class	Cys	Glut	CD	GD	CG	GG
Carbonyls			735.9	399.5	31.5	26.5
Furans			19.2	15.9	88.4	159.0
Thiazoles	488.2	72.6	30.0	50.1	125.9	38.3
Thiophenes	47.8	2.5	219.0	339.6	400.8	141.8
Pyridines	2.1		501.1	1219.0		
Pyrroles	23.7					
Pyrazines					117.6	31.6
Poly-*S*-compounds	3220.8	740.7	1373.1	537.0	204.6	7.0
Total	3782.6	815.8	2879.6	2561.1	968.8	404.2

[a]Model reaction systems: Cys, cysteine alone;[22] Glut, glutathione alone;[22] CD, cysteine reacted with 2,4-decadienal;[23] GD, glutathione reacted with 2,4-decadienal;[23] CG, cysteine reacted with glucose;[24] GG, glutathione reacted with glucose.[24]

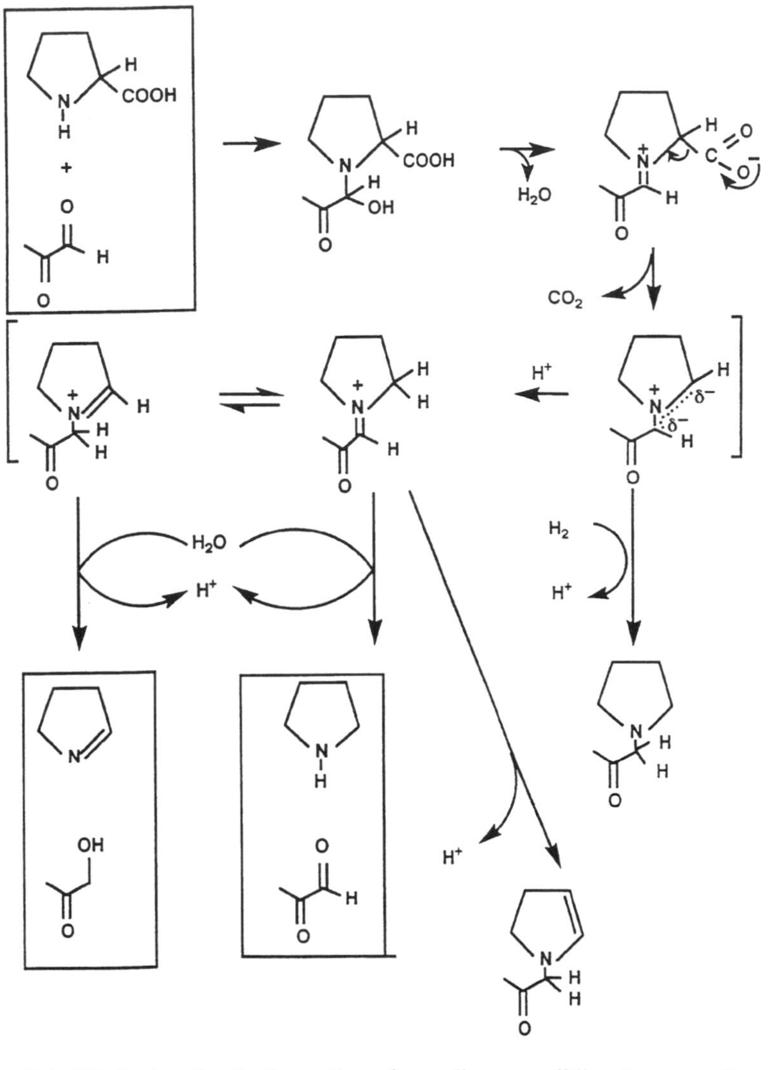

Figure 2.4. Mechanism for the formation of pyrroline, pyrrolidine, 1-acetonylpyrrolidine and 1-acetonyl-2-pyrroline. (Reprinted with permission from Ref. 25. Copyright 1985, American Chemical Society)

promoted but the generation of other sulfur-containing compounds was depressed, especially in the glutathione–glucose system.

PROLINE-SPECIFIC COMPOUNDS

The volatiles formed from the reaction between proline and simple sugars have been analyzed thoroughly by Tressl *et al.*[25-27] The reactions used equimolar amounts of proline, which was heated separately, with glyceraldehyde, erythrose, arabinose, glucose and rhamnose at 150 °C for 30 minutes. Pyrrolidines, piperidines, pyrrolizines and azepines were identified as proline-specific Maillard reaction products.

Pyrrolidines and Piperidines

The formation of pyrrolines and pyrrolidines could be explained as a result of the interaction between proline with α-dicarbonyls such as pyruvaldehyde as shown in Figure 2.4. Dehydration of the interaction compounds led to the formation of an iminium carboxylate intermediate which further decarboxylated and protonated to the formation of the ylide or imminium ion. These ylides are important key intermediates in the formation of proline-specific compounds. Hydration and reduction of these intermediates lead to the formation of 1-pyrroline or pyrrolidine and 1-acetonylpyrrolidine.

Among the pyrrolines identified by Tressl *et al.*[28] 2-acetyl-1-pyrroline has an intense cracker-like odor. This compound has been shown to be an impact compound in the crust of wheat bread.[29] The pyrrolidines possess a pleasant cereal or sesame-like aroma. On the other hand, the piperidines do not have specific characteristic aromas. The piperidines, however, are easily transformed to tetrahydropyridines upon dehydration, and these tetrahydropyridines possess bready, cracker-like aromas with a very low flavor threshold, in the ppb range. The formation of piperidines was assumed via ring enlargement of the pyrrolidines, as shown in Figure 2.5.

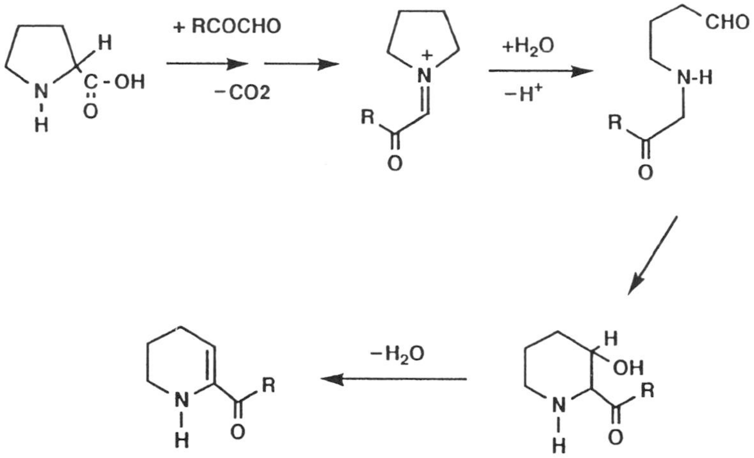

Figure 2.5. Proposed mechanism for the formation of piperidines and tetrahydropyridines from proline. (Adapted with permission from Ref. 28. Copyright 1981, Walter de Gruyter)

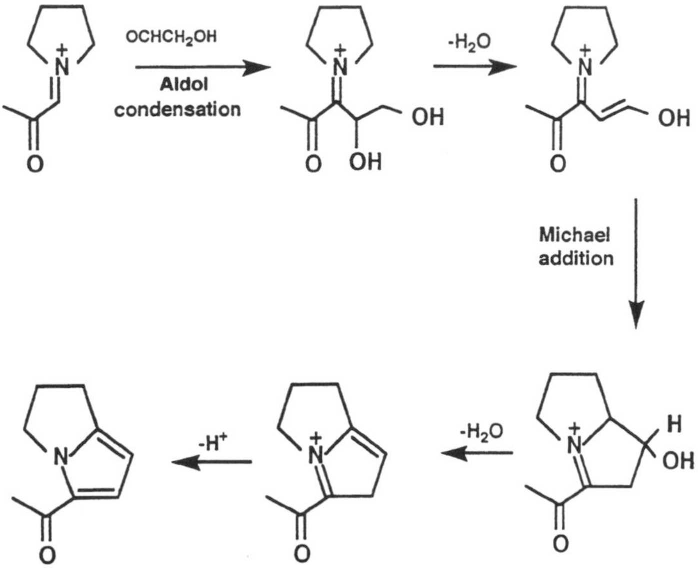

Figure 2.6. Proposed mechanism for the formation of pyrrolizines from proline. (Adapted and reprinted with permission from Ref 26. Copyright 1985, American Chemical Society)

2,3-Dihydro-1*H*-pyrrolizines

Pyrrolizines possess smoky and roasty aromas. Three pyrrolizines have been identified by Shigematsu *et al.*[30] Tressl's group identified another 18 pyrrolizines in their study.[26] The proposed mechanism for the formation of pyrrolizines (Figure 2.6) was initiated with interaction of proline and dicarbonyl to produce iminium carboxylate which decarboxylated to form an ylide. This ylide reacted further with an α-hydroxycarbonyl to form an intermediate which underwent dehydration to form the more stable conjugated product. This conjugated intermediate was transformed to a fused ring compound through Michael addition. Dehydration and tautomerism were followed after a ring closure to the more thermodynamically stable pyrrolizines.

Although 2,3-dihydro-1*H*-pyrrolizines were mainly identified in systems containing proline, several derivatives of 2,3-dihydro-1*H*-pyrrolizine have been reported in the Maillard reaction of sucrose with threonine or serine[31] as well as the reaction of xylose with lysine.[32]

Cyclopent[b]azepine-8(1*H*)-ones

Tressl's group[27] proposed that azepines, obtained during the reaction of proline with monosaccharide, might be derived from the reaction of proline

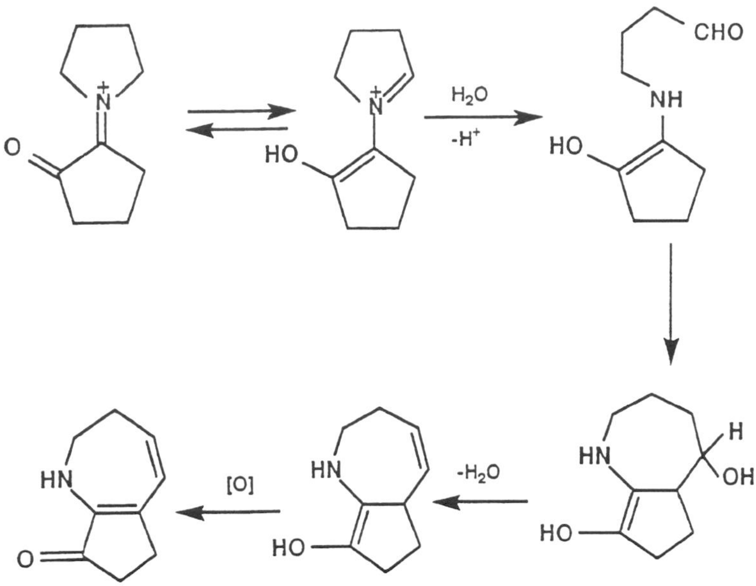

Figure 2.7. Proposed mechanism for the formation of azepines from proline. (Adapted and reprinted with permission from Ref 27. Copyright 1989, American Chemical Society)

with pentenolone. They found that the reaction of proline and pentenolone increased the azepines formation a thousandfold. The mechanistic pathway for the formation of azepines is shown in Figure 2.7. The reaction begins with the formation of a Schiff's base between proline and pentenolone to form 1-pyrrolidinylcyclopentenones. The enol form of 1-pyrrolidinylcyclopentenones undergoes a pyrrole ring opening and cyclization to form a larger seven-member fused ring. The formation of azepines is accomplished by further dehydration and oxidation.

METHIONINE-SPECIFIC COMPOUNDS

Maillard products identified in methionine–reducing sugar model experiments result predominantly from the Strecker aldehyde (methional) and methylmercaptan, respectively. Figure 2.8 summarizes methionine-specific compounds reported by Tressl et al.[19] Heterocyclic compounds containing a methylthioethyl or methylthiopropyl side chain such as 2-(2-methylthioethyl)-4,5-dimethyloxazole and 2-(3-methylthiopropyl)-5,6-dimethylpyrazine are most interesting. Similar compounds such as 2-(2-methylthioethyl)-4,5-dimethyl-3-oxazoline and 2-(4-methylthiobutyl)-3,5,6-trimethylpyrazine have been reported by Hartman and Ho[33] in the reaction of methionine with 2,3-

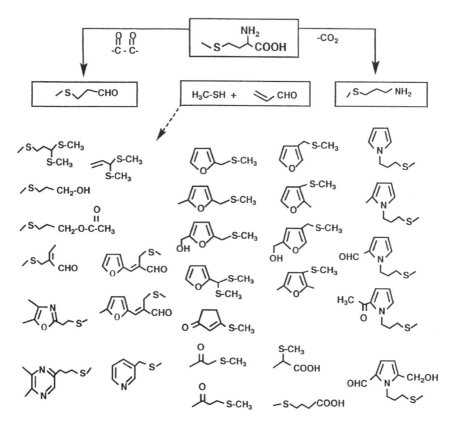

Figure 2.8. Strecker degradation products identified in methionine/reducing sugar model systems. (Reprinted with permission from Ref. 19. Copyright 1989, American Chemical Society)

butanedione. The formation of 2-(2-methylthioethyl)-4,5-dimethyloxazole and its oxazoline analog can be explained by the mechanism set forth by Rizzi,[34] as shown in Figure 2.9.[33]

ASPARAGINE-SPECIFIC COMPOUNDS

Shu and Lawrence[35] reported the identification of 3,5-dimethyl-6-ethyl-2(1*H*)-pyrazinone, 3,6-dimethyl-5-ethyl-2(1*H*)-pyrazinone, 3,5,6-trimethyl-2(1*H*)-pyr-azinone and 3-methyl-5,6-diethyl-2(1*H*)-pyrazinone as asparagine-specific Maillard products from the reaction of asparagine and monosaccharides. The formation of this group of compounds has been proposed to be a condensation process between α-dicarbonyl and alanine amide, as shown in

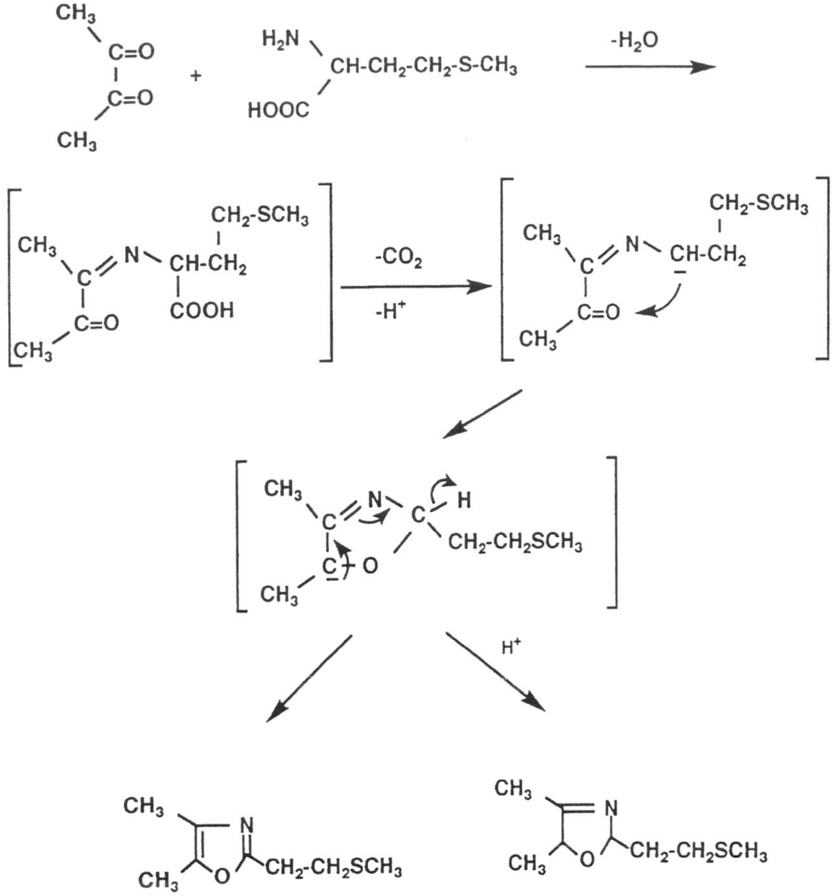

Figure 2.9. Formation of 2-(2-methylthioethyl)-4,5-dimethyloxazole and 2-(2-methylthioethyl)-4,5-dimethyl-3-oxazoline from the reaction of methionine and 2,3-butanedione. (Reprinted with permission from Ref. 33. Copyright 1984, Academic Press)

Figure 2.10. The latter is generated from asparagine via cyclic imide and isoasparagine by decarboxylation.

HISTIDINE-SPECIFIC COMPOUNDS

By reacting histidine with glucose under the conditions of roasting and autoclaving, Gi and Baltes[36] identified 2-acetyl- and 2-propionyl-pyrido[3,4-d]imidazole along with their corresponding tetrahydropyrido derivatives as histidine-specific compounds. 2-Acetyl-pyrido[3,4-d]imidazole was also formed by heating glucose with tuna fish. The proposed mechanism for the formation

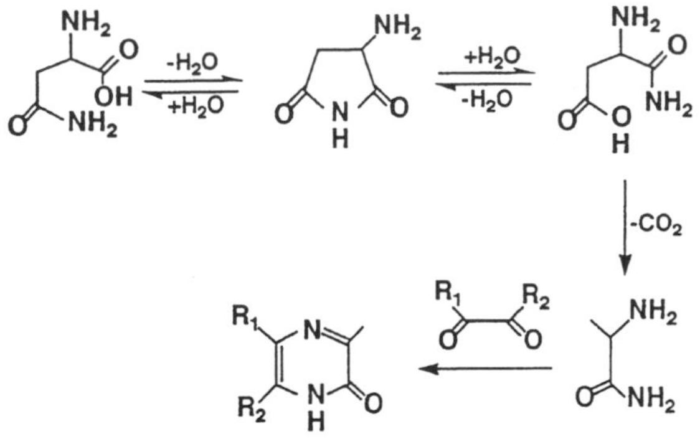

Figure 2.10. Mechanism for the formation of 3-methyl-2(1H)-pyrazinone from the reaction of asparagine and glucose

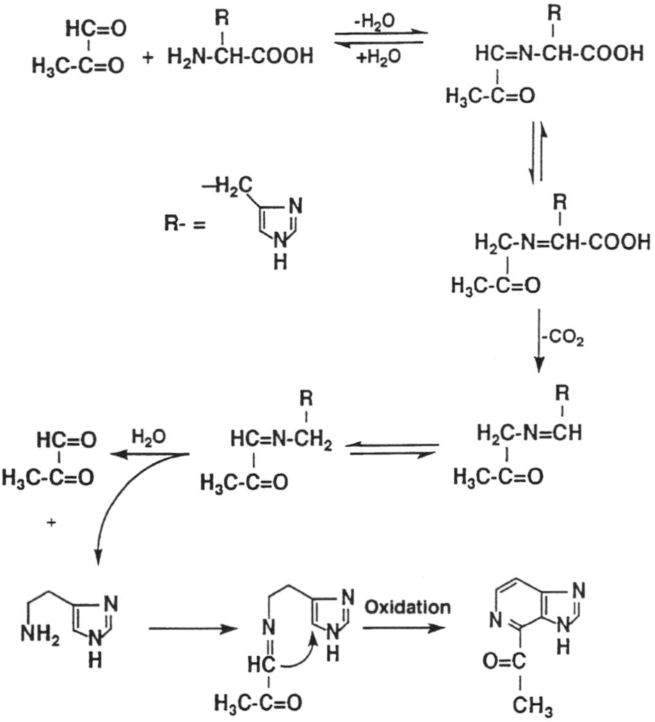

Figure 2.11. Mechanism proposed for the formation of 2-acetyl-pyrido[3,4-*d*]-imidazole via Strecker degradation of histidine with pyruvic aldehyde. (Reprinted with permission from Ref. 36. Copyright 1994, American Chemical Society)

Table 2.4. The amount of 1-alkyl-2(1*H*)-pyrazinones identified from the reaction of glucose with peptides

Compounds	Amount (mc/mole peptide)				
	di-Gly	tri-Gly	tetra-Gly	Gly–Leu	Leu–Gly
1,6-Dimethyl-2(1*H*)-pyrazinone	323.00	119.35	422.35		
1,5-Dimethyl-2(1*H*)-pyrazinone	t[a]	t	1.37		
1,5,6-Trimethyl-2(1*H*)-pyrazinone	t	2.85	0.57		
1-Methyl-3-isobutyl-2(1*H*)-pyrazinone				351.41	433.59
1-Isopentyl-2(1*H*)-pyrazinone				185.58	129.95
1,6-Dimethyl-3-isobutyl-2(1*H*)-pyrazinone				1629.69	1234.09
1,5,6-Trimethyl-3-isobutyl-2(1*H*)-pyrazinone				84.17	83.54

[a]t = trace.

of 2-acetyl-pyrido[3,4-*d*]imidazole via Strecker degradation of histidine with pyruvic aldehyde is shown in Figure 2.11.

PEPTIDES-SPECIFIC COMPOUNDS

The generation of peptide-specific aroma compounds, 1-alkyl-2(1*H*)-pyrazinones, has been reported in the reaction of glucose with diglycine, triglycine, tetraglycine, Gly–Leu and Leu–Gly.[37-39] Table 2.4 shows the type and amount of 1-alkyl-2(1*H*)-pyrazinones identified in these reactions. These 1-alkyl-2(1*H*)-pyrazinones were generated by the direct condensation of dicarbonyl with dipeptide, followed by the decarboxylation reaction as shown in Figure 2.12.

MAJOR CLASSES OF MAILLARD REACTION AROMA COMPOUNDS

STRECKER ALDEHYDES

Strecker degradation is one of the most important reactions leading to the final aroma compounds in the Maillard reaction. It involves the initial Schiff base formation of an α-dicarbonyl compound with an amino acid. After rearrangement, decarboxylation and hydrolysis, the α-amino carbonyl compound and Strecker aldehyde are generated. Figure 2.13 shows the mechanism for the Strecker degradation. α-Amino carbonyl compounds are precursors of the most important flavor compounds, pyrazines. Many Strecker aldehydes are also significant food flavors. For examples, methional is the impact compound of potato products and isovaldehyde is significant to the

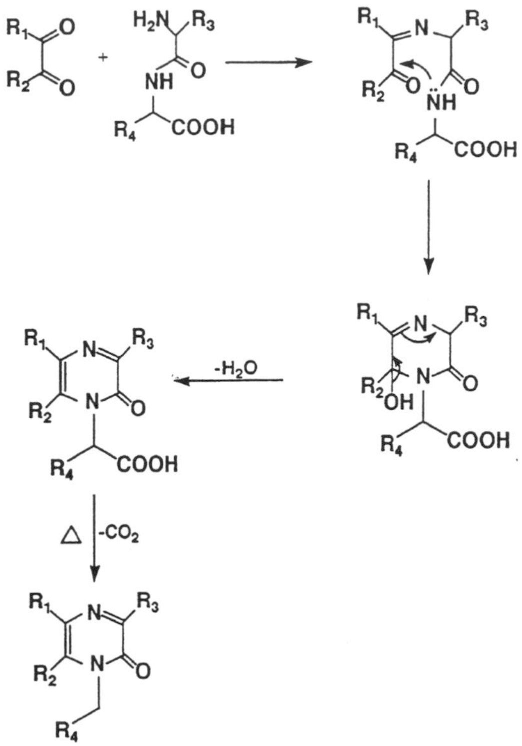

Figure 2.12. Mechanism for the formation of 1-alkyl-2(1*H*)-pyrazinones from the reaction of dipeptide with α-dicarbonyl

flavor of cocoa. Table 2.5 lists sensory properties of selected Strecker aldehydes.[40]

PYRAZINES

Pyrazines have been recognized as important flavor components of a large number of cooked, roasted and toasted foods. The occurrence of alkylpyrazines in foods has been extensively reviewed.[41-42] The alkylpyrazines generally have nutty and roasted aromas. These unique and desirable sensory properties make pyrazines essential to the food industry.

The most direct route for pyrazine formation results from the condensation of two molecules of α-amino ketone. The α-amino ketone could be generated by the interaction of α-dicarbonyls and α-amino acids through Strecker degradation. On the other hand, α-amino ketone may also be produced by the reaction of free ammonia with α-hydroxyketones. Both α-dicarbonyls and α-hydroxyketones are the retro-aldolization products of

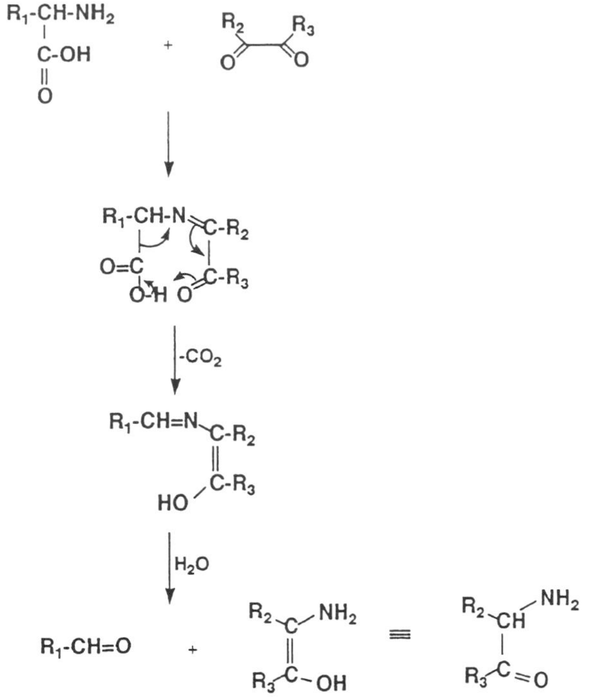

Figure 2.13. Mechanism for the Strecker degradation of amino acids

Table 2.5. Sensory properties of some Strecker aldehydes

Strecker aldehyde	Amino acid	Odor properties
Acetaldehyde	Alanine	Pungent, ethereal, green, sweet
Isobutyraldehyde	Valine	Extremely diffusive, pungent, green, in extreme dilution almost pleasant, fruity, banana-like
2-Methylbutanal	Isoleucine	Powerful, but in extreme dilution almost fruity — 'fermented' with a peculiar note resembling that of roasted cocoa or coffee
Isovaldehyde	Leucine	Very powerful, acrid-pungent. In extreme dilution fruity, rather pleasant
Methional	Methionine	Powerful onion–meat-like, potato-like
Phenylacetaldehyde	Phenylalanine	Very powerful, pungent, floral and sweet

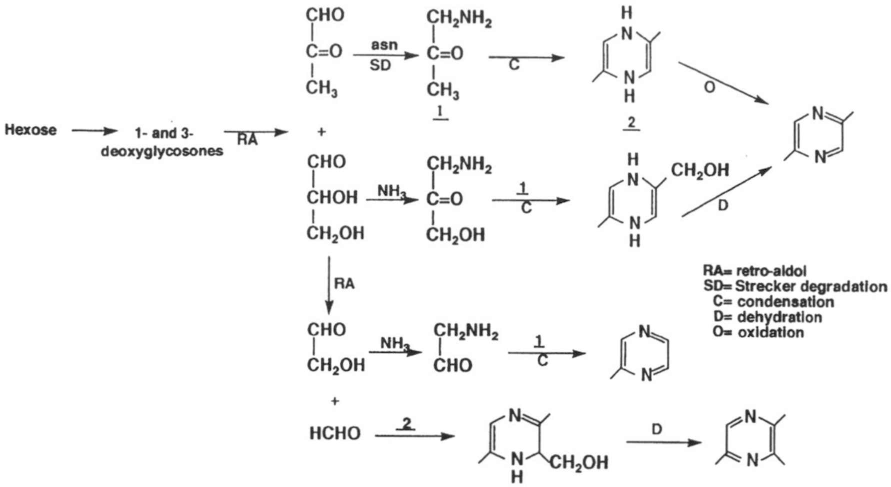

Figure 2.14. Formation of pyrazines from hexose and asparagine. (Reprinted with permission from Ref. 43. Copyright 1994, American Chemical Society)

1-deoxyosone or 3-deoxyosone. A representative mechanism for the formation of pyrazines from the reaction of hexose with asparagine proposed by Weenen *et al.*[43] is shown in Figure 2.14. By reacting ^{13}C-labeled glucose (1-^{13}C-glucose and 2-^{13}C-glucose) with asparagine, the ^{13}C incorporation in pyrazines obtained was in agreement with retro-aldolization of the intermediate deoxyglucosones as the main cleavage mechanism.[43] Both 1- and 3-deoxyglucosone play an approximately equal role in the formation of the alkylpyrazines.

Recently, the contribution of amino and amide nitrogen atoms to pyrazine formation has been investigated.[44] When the ^{15}N isotope labeled at the amide side chain of glutamine was reacted with glucose at 180 °C in dry or aqueous systems, more than half of the nitrogen atoms in the alkylpyrazine ring consisted of ^{15}N atoms that came from the amide chain of glutamine. Table 2.6 shows the relative contribution of amide nitrogens to pyrazine formation in both dry and aqueous systems. These observations demonstrated that deamidation of glutamine and asparagine did happen under the conditions of Maillard reaction and it could participate in the pyrazine formation. A similar study also showed that both the α- and ε-amino groups of lysine were involved in the pyrazine formation.[45]

PYRIDINES

Many alkylpyridines and acylpyridins have been reported in coffee, barley and meat.[46,47] Some pyridines have pleasant odors; however, most pyridines have

Table 2.6. Relative contributions of amide nitrogens to pyrazine formation in the reaction of labeled glutamine–amide–^{15}N with glucose

Pyrazine compound	Contribution of amide nitrogen (%)	
	Dry system	Aqueous system
Pyrazine	76.76	82.26
Methylpyrazine	79.81	74.03
2,5- and 2,6-Dimethylpyrazine	62.19	52.53
Ethylpyrazine	73.55	73.09
2,3-Dimethylpyrazine	68.43	68.63
Vinylpyrazine	79.17	93.89
2-Ethyl-5-methylpyrazine	68.87	
2-Vinyl-6-methylpyrazine		61.75

green, bitter, astringent, roasted, burnt, vegetable pungent or phenolic properties.[48,49] In general, alkylpyridines possess less desirable flavor[40] whereas acylpyridines have more pleasant aromas. For example, 2-acetylpyridine has a cracker-type aroma.[50] The pyridine formation pathway involves the condensation of aldehydes, ketones or α,β-unsaturated carbonyl compounds with ammonia which is degraded from amino acids.

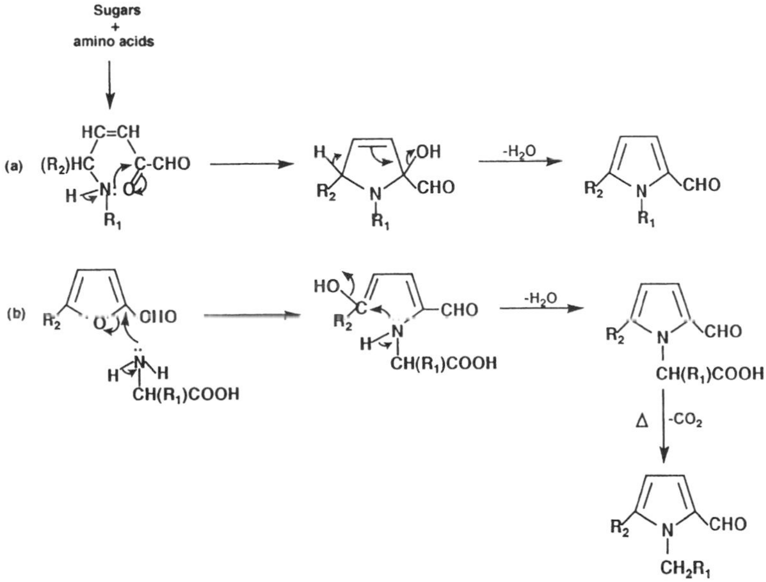

Figure 2.15. Formation of 1-alkyl-2-formalpyrroles from sugars or further and α-amino acids. (Reproduced from Ref. 8 by permission of Ellis Horwood Publishers)

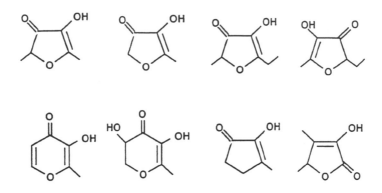

Figure 2.16. Structures of selected 'browned flavor' compounds

PYRROLES

Pyrroles tend to contribute baked cereal-type or smoky notes and have been reported in various heated foods, especially in coffee.[40,51] A large number of pyrroles, mainly 2-acylpyrroles, were identified in several model systems including glucose–ammonia[52] and lactose–casein.[53] Mechanisms for the formation of 1-alkyl-2-formylpyrroles from sugars or furfural and amino acids have been suggested, as shown in Figure 2.15.[8]

FURANS, FURANONES AND PYRANONES

Furans are formed by thermal degradation of carbohydrates and from the Maillard reaction during food processing. They are present in nearly all food aromas.[54] Alkylfurans usually possess sweet, burnt and pungent odors. If the substituents contain aldehyde, ketone or alcohol functional groups, they are usually burnt and caramellic.[40]

Many furanones and pyranones containing the α-diketone or β-diketone structures are referred to as 'browned flavors'. It has been postulated by Hodge[55] that the caramel-like odor was a function of a specific feature, which is a planar enol–carbonyl substructure of cyclic dicarbonyl compounds. Some examples of compounds in this category are shown in Figure 2.16. These compounds are usually formed by cyclization and dehydration of 1-deoxy-osones or 3-deoxyosones.

OXAZOLES

Oxazoles and oxazolines are heterocyclic compounds containing both oxygen and nitrogen atoms. They possess potent sensory qualities at low concentration and are generally described as green, nutty and sweet. The occurrence of oxazoles has been reported in cocoa,[56] coffee,[57] meat products,[58] roasted barley,[59] baked potato,[60] roasted peanuts,[61] cocoa butter[62] and french fried potato.[63]

The first oxazoline, 2,4,5-trimethyl-3-oxazoline, was reported by Chang *et al.*[64] in the volatiles of boiled beef. Mussinan *et al.*[65] identified oxazolines but no oxazoles in their beef system. On the other hand, Peterson *et al.*[66] reported that in the volatiles of beef stew, both 2,4,5-trimethyloxazole and 2,4,5-trimethyl-3-oxazoline were present and the relative size of the gas chromatographic peak associated with 2,4,5-trimethyloxazole was medium whereas that for 2,4,5-trimethyl-3-oxazoline was extra large.

Mussinan *et al.*[65] has suggested that 2,4,5-trimethyl-3-oxazoline can form in heated meat systems by the thermal interaction and rearrangement of the compounds, ammonia, acetaldehyde and acetoin. Rizzi[34] and Ho and Hartman[67] identified the oxazoles and 3-oxazolines in the Strecker degradation of amino acids such as valine, alanine and cysteine with 2,3-butanedione. The mechanism is similar to that shown in Figure 2.9 for the formation of 2-(2-methylthioethyl)-4,5-dimethyloxazole and its oxazoline analog in the reaction of methionine with 2,3-butanedione.

LIPID–MAILLARD INTERACTIONS IN THE FORMATION OF AROMA COMPOUNDS

The oxidation of lipids is as important as the Maillard reaction for the formation of flavor in cooked foods. However, these reactions do not occur in isolation; all foods, whether of animal or vegetable origin, comprise a complex mixture of components, including lipids, sugars and amino acids. Thus, cooking of foods would be expected to facilitate interaction between the Maillard and lipid oxidation pathways.[68] In recent years, the role of lipid–Maillard interactions in the formation of aroma compounds has been investigated both in foods and in model systems. The subject has recently been reviewed.[69]

EFFECT OF LIPID OXIDATION PRODUCTS ON PYRAZINE FORMATION

A typical reaction scheme of the involvement of lipid-derived carbonyl compounds in the formation of pyrazines through a Maillard-type reaction was shown in a model system[70] using hydroxyacetone, ammonium acetate and different aliphatic aldehydes. With ammonium acetate used as an ammonia source, which represents a protein or an amino acid, hydroxyacetate represents an α-dicarbonyl compound from the Maillard reaction and aldehydes are typical lipid oxidation products. The pentyl- or hexyl-substituted pyrazines

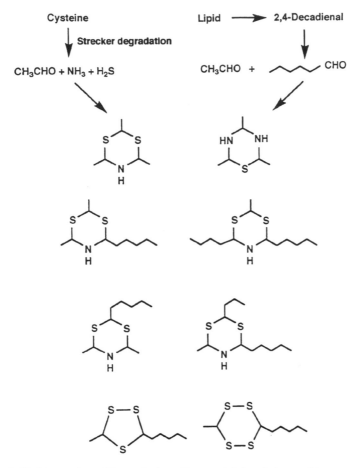

Figure 2.17. Formation of long-chain sulfur-containing heterocyclic compounds from lipid-derived aldehydes

were formed from the model systems with the pentanal and hexanal, respectively.

These long-chain alkyl-substituted pyrazines have so far been identified in a few food systems, including fried chicken,[71] baked potato,[60] and french fries.[72]

EFFECT OF LIPID OXIDATION PRODUCTS ON SULFUR-CONTAINING COMPOUND FORMATION

Lipid-derived aldehydes participated in the formation of long-chain sulfur-containing heterocyclic compounds in the Maillard reaction when cysteine or cysteine-containing peptides were present. In a model system mimicking the

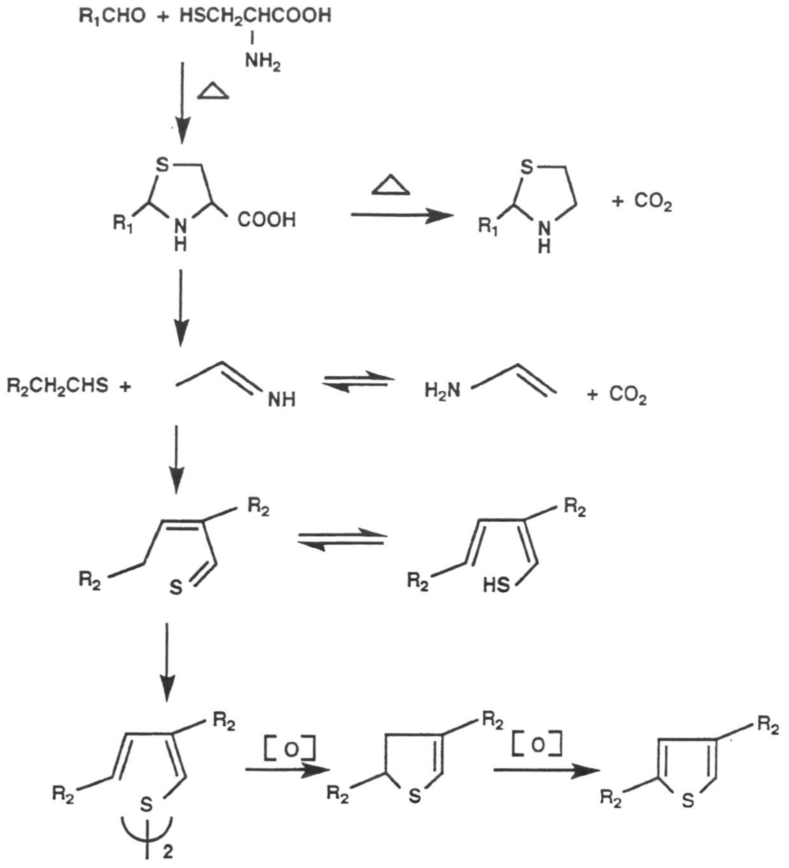

Figure 2.18. Formation of 2,4-dialkylthiophenes from lipid-derived aldehydes. (Adapted from Ref. 75. Reproduced by permission of Elsevier Science)

contribution of lipids to the formation of meat flavors, Zhang and Ho[23] conducted an interaction of 2,4-decadienal, an important oxidation product of linoleic acid, with cysteine. Figure 2.17 shows the formation pathway for the selected alkyl-substituted sulfur-containing compounds formed in these systems. Except for 3-methyl-5-pentyl-1,2,4-trithiolane identified in fried chicken,[71] none of the other long-chain alkyl-substituted sulfur-containing compounds shown in Figure 2.17 have ever been identified in foods.

One important class of cysteine-specific aroma compounds not discussed in the previously section is thiazoles. The potential for thiazole derivatives as flavorants is evident from the work of Stoll *et al.*,[73] who found that the strong nut-like odor of a cocoa extract was due to a trace amount of 4-methyl-5-

vinylthiazole. Since then, numerous thiazoles have been identified in food flavors.

Several alkylthiazoles identified in fried chicken and french fried potato flavors have long-chain alkyl substituents on the thiazole ring.[72] They include 2-pentyl-4,5-dimethylthiazole, 2-hexyl-4,5-dimethylthiazole, 2-heptyl-4,5-dimethylthiazole, 2-heptyl-4-ethylthiazole and 2-octyl-4,5-dimethylthiazole. Very recently, Farmer and Mottram[68] reported the identification of very long-chain ($^{13}C-^{15}C$) alkyl-substituted thiazoles in beef and chicken meat. These thiazoles with the long alkyl chain in the 2 position almost certainly arise from the reaction of dicarbonyl compounds (from sugar degradation), H_2S and NH_3 (from the Strecker of cysteine) and a long-chain aldehyde derived from lipid oxidation, as described by Takken *et al.*[74]

Another cysteine-specific reaction with lipid-derived aldehydes may lead to the formation of 2,4-dialkylthiophenes, as reported recently by Rizzi *et al.*[75] The mechanism is shown in Figure 2.18. Five different 2,4-dialkylthiophenes from the corresponding aldehydes with cysteine were characterized.[73] In an independent study, 2,4-dibutylthiophene was identified in the reaction of 2,4-decadienal with cysteine.[23]

REFERENCES

1. C. Eriksson, *Maillard Reactions in Foods*, Pergamon Press, Oxford, 1981.
2. G. W. Waller and M. S. Feather, *The Maillard Reaction in Foods and Nutrition*, ACS Symposium Series 215, American Chemical Society, Washington, D.C., 1983.
3. M. Fujimaki, M. Namiki and H. Kato, *Amino-Carbonyl Reactions in Food and Biological Systems*, Kodansha, Ltd, Tokyo, 1986.
4. P. A. Finot, H. U. Aeschbacher, R. F. Hurrell and R. Liardon, *The Maillard Reaction in Food Processing, Human Nutrition and Physiology*, Birkhauser Verlag, Basel, 1990.
5. T. H. Parliment, R. J. McGorrin and C.-T. Ho, *Thermal Generation of Aromas*, ACS Symposium Series 409, American Chemical Society, Washington, D.C., 1989.
6. T. H. Parliment, M. J. Morello and R. J. McGorrin, *Thermally Generated Flavors*, ACS Symposium Series 543, American Chemical Society, Washington, D.C., 1994.
7. T. H. Parliment, Thermal generation of aromas, an overview, in *Thermal Generation of Aromas* (eds. T. H. Parliment, R. J. McGorrin and C.-T. Ho). ACS Symposium Series 409, American Chemical Society, Washington, D.C., 1989, pp. 2–11.
8. G. Vernin and C. Parkanyi, Mechanisms of formation of heterocyclic compounds in Maillard and pyrolysis reactions, in *The Chemistry of Heterocyclic Flavoring and Aroma Compounds* (ed. G. Vernin), Ellis Horwood Publishers, Chichester, 1982, pp. 151–207.
9. I. Blank, A. Sen and W. Grosch, Potent odorants of the roasted powder and brew of Arabica coffee, *Z. Lebensm. Unters. Forsch.*, **195**, 239–45 (1992).
10. P. Schieberle and W. Grosch, Bread flavor, in *Thermal Generation of Aromas* (eds. T. H. Parliment, R. J. McGorrin and C.-T. Ho), American Chemical Society, Washington, D. C. 1989, pp. 258–67.

11. P. Schieberle and W. Grosch, Potent odorants of rye crust. Differences from the crumb and wheat bread crust, *Z. Lebensm. Unters. Forsch.*, **198**, 292–6 (1994).

12. H. Guth and W. Grosch, 12-Methyltridecanal, a species-specific odorant of stewed beef, *Lebensm. Wiss. und-Technol.*, **26**, 171–7 (1993).

13. C. Cerny and W. Grosch, Evaluation of potent odorants in roasted beef by extract dilution analysis, *Z. Lebensm. Unters. Forsch.*, **194**, 322–5 (1992).

14. P. Schieberle, Studies on the flavour of roasted white sesame seeds, in *Progress in Flavour Precursor Studies* (ed. P. Schreier and P. Winterhalter), Allured Publishing Co., Carol Stream, 1993, pp. 343–60.

15. P. Schieberle, Primary odorants in popcorn, *J. Agric. Food Chem.*, **39**, 1141–44 (1991).

16. M. Boelens, L. M. van der Linde, P. J. de Valois, H. M. van Dort and H. J. Takken, Organic sulfur compounds from fatty aldehydes, hydrogen sulfide, thiols and ammonia as flavor constituents, *J. Agric. Food Chem.*, **22**, 1071–6 (1974).

17. C. K. Shu, M. L. Hagedorn, B. D. Mookherjee and C.-T. Ho, Volatile components of the thermal degradation of cysteine in water, *J. Agric. Food Chem.*, **33**, 438–42 (1985).

18. C. K. Shu, M. L. Hagedorn, B. D. Mookherjee and C.-T. Ho, pH effect on the volatile components in the thermal degradation of cysteine, *J. Agric. Food Chem.*, **33**, 442–6 (1985).

19. R. Tressl, B. Helak, N. Martin and E. Kersten, Formation of amino acid specific Maillard products and their contribution to thermally generated aromas, in *Thermal Generation of Aromas* (eds. T. H. Parliment, R. J. McGorrin and C.-T. Ho), ACS Symposium Series 409, American Chemical Society, Washington, D.C., 1989, pp. 156–71.

20. W. Holscher and H. Steinhart, Formation pathways for primary roasted coffee aroma compounds, in *Thermally Generated Flavors* (eds. T. H. Parliment, M. J. Morello and R. J. McGorrin), ACS Symposium Series 543, American Chemical Society, Washington, D.C., 1994, pp. 206–17.

21. D. A. M. van den Ouweland and H. G. Peer, Components contributing to beef flavor. Volatile compounds produced by the reaction of 4-hydroxy-5-methyl-3(2*H*)-furanone and its thionanalog with hydrogen sulfide, *J. Agric. Food Chem.*, **23**, 501–5 (1975).

22. Y. Zhang, M. Chien and C.-T. Ho, Comparison of the volatile compounds obtained from thermal degradation of cysteine and glutathione, *J. Agric. Food Chem.*, **36**, 992–6 (1988).

23. Y. Zhang and C.-T. Ho, Volatile compounds formed from thermal interaction of 2,4-decadienal with cysteine and glutathione, *J. Agric. Food Chem.*, **37**, 1016–20 (1989).

24. Y. Zhang and C.-T. Ho, Comparison of the volatile compounds formed from the thermal reaction of glucose with cysteine and glutathione, *J. Agric. Food Chem.*, **39**, 760–3 (1991).

25. R. Tressl, D. Rewicki, B. Helak and H. Kampershroer, Formation of pyrrolidines and piperidines on heating L-proline with reducing sugars, *J. Agric. Food Chem.*, **33**, 924–8 (1985).

26. R. Tressl, D. Rewicki, B. Helak, H. Kampershroer and N. Martin, Formation of 2,3-dihydro-1*H*-pyrrolizines as proline specific Maillard products, *J. Agric. Food Chem.*, **33**, 919–23 (1985).

27. R. Tressl, B. Helak, H. Koppler and D. Rewicki, Formation of 2-(1-pyrrolidinyl)-2-cyclopentenones and cyclopent(b)azepin-8(1*H*)-one as proline specific Maillard products, *J. Agric. Food Chem.*, **33**, 1132–7 (1985).

28. R. Tressl, K. G. Grünewald and B. Helak, Formation of flavour components from proline and hydroxyproline with glucose and maltose and their importance to food flavour, in *Flavour '81* (ed. P. Schreier), Walter de Gruyter, Berlin, 1981, pp. 397–416.

29. P. Schieberle, Formation of 2-acetyl-1-pyrroline and other important flavor compounds in wheat bread crust, in *Thermal Generation of Aromas* (eds. T. H. Parliment, R. J. McGorrin and C.-T. Ho), ACS Symposium Series 409, American Chemical Society, Washington, D.C. 1989, pp. 268–75.

30. H. Shigematsu, S. Shibata, T. Kurata, H. Kato and M. Fujimaki, 5-Acetyl-2,3-dihydro-1*H*-pyrrolizines and 5,6,7,8-tetrahydroindilizin-8-ones, odor constituents formed on heating L-proline with D-glucose, *J. Agric. Food Chem.*, **23**, 233–7 (1975).

31. W. Baltes and G. Bochmann, Model reactions on roast aroma formation: III. Mass spectrometric identification of pyrroles from the reaction of serine and threonine with sucrose under the conditions of coffee roasting, *Z. Lebensm. Unter. Forsch.*, **184**, 478–4 (1987).

32. J. M. Ames and A. Apriyantono, Effect of pH on the volatile compounds formed in a xylose–lysine model system, in *Thermally Generated Flavors* (eds. T. H. Parliment, M. J. Morello and R. J. McGorrin), ACS Symposium Series 543, American Chemical Society, Washington, D.C., 1994, pp. 228–39.

33. G. J. Hartman and C.-T. Ho, Volatile products of the reaction of sulfur-containing amino acids with 2,3-butanedione, *Lebensm. -Wiss. u. -Technol.*, **17**, 171–4 (1984).

34. G. P. Rizzi, The formation of tetramethylpyrazine and 2-isopropyl-4,5-dimethyl-3-oxazoline in the Strecker degradation of DL-valine with 2,3-butanedione, *J. Org. Chem.*, **34**, 2002–4 (1969).

35. C. K. Shu and B. M. Lawrence, Presented at the 208th National Meeting of the American Chemical Society, Washington, D.C., 1994.

36. U. S. Gi and W. Baltes, Pyridoimidazoles, histidine-specific reaction products, in *Thermally Generated Flavors* (eds. T. H. Parliment, M. J. Morello and R. J. McGorrin), ACS Symposium Series 543, American Chemical Society, Washington, D.C., 1994, pp. 263–9.

37. Y. C. Oh, C. K. Shu and C.-T. Ho, Formation of novel 2(1*H*)-pyrazinones as peptide-specific Maillard reaction products, *J. Agric. Food Chem.*, **40**, 118–21 (1992).

38. C.-T. Ho, Y. C. Oh, Y. Zhang and C. K. Shu, Peptides as flavor precursors in model Maillard reactions, in *Flavor Precursors, Thermal and Enzymatic Conversions* (eds. R. Teranishi, G. R. Takeoka and M. Güntert), ACS Symposium Series 490, American Chemical Society, Washington, D.C., 1992, pp. 193–202.

39. H. V. Izzo and C.-T. Ho, Peptide specific Maillard reaction products: a new pathway for flavor chemistry, *Trends Food Sci. Technol.*, **3**, 253–7 (1992).

40. S. Fors, Sensory properties of volatile Maillard reaction products and related compounds, in *The Maillard Reaction in Foods and Nutrition* (eds. G. R. Waller and M. S. Feather), ACS Symposium Series 215, American Chemical Society, Washington, D.C., 1983, pp. 185–286.

41. J. A. Maga, Pyrazines in foods: an update, *CRC Crit. Rev. Food Sci. Nutr.*, **16**, 1–48 (1982).

42. J. A. Maga, Pyrazines update, *Food Rev. Interact*, **8**, 479–558 (1992).

43. H. Weenen, S. B. Tjan, P. J. de Valois and H. Vonk, Mechanism of pyrazine formation, in *Thermally Generated Flavors* (eds T. H. Parliment, M. J. Morello and R. J. McGorrin), ACS Symposium Series 543, American Chemical Society, Washington, D.C., 1994, pp. 142–57.

44. H. I. Hwang, T. G. Hartman, R. T. Rosen and C.-T. Ho, Formation of pyrazines from the Maillard reaction of glucose and glutamine-amide-^{15}N, *J. Agric. Food Chem.*, **41**, 2112–14 (1993).

45. H. I. Hwang, T. G. Hartman, R. T. Rosen, J. Lech and C.-T. Ho, Formation of pyrazines from the Maillard reaction of glucose and lysine-α-amine-^{15}N, *J. Agric. Food Chem.*, **42**, 1000–4 (1994).

46. D. S. Mottram, Meat, in *Volatile Compounds in Foods and Beverages* (ed. H. Maarse), Marcel Dekker, New York, 1991, p. 107.

47. K. Suyama and S. Adachi, Origin of alkyl-substituted pyridines in food flavor: formation of pyridines from the reaction of alkanals with amino acids, *J. Agric. Food Chem.*, **28**, 546–9 (1980).

48. J. A. Maga, Pyridines in food, *J. Agric. Food Chem.*, **29**, 895–8 (1981).

49. A. O. Pittet and D. E. Hruza, Comparative study of flavor properties of thiazole derivatives, *J. Agric. Food Chem.*, **22**, 264–9 (1974).

50. R. G. Buttery, R. M. Seifert, D. G. Guadagni and L. C. Ling, Characterization of additional volatile components of tomato, *J. Agric. Food Chem.*, **19**, 524–9 (1971).

51. I. Flament, Coffee, cocoa, and tea, in *Volatile Compounds in Foods and Beverages* (ed. H. Maarse), Marcel Dekker, New York, 1991, pp. 617–69.

52. T. Shibamoto, T. Akiyama, M. Sakaguchi, Y. Enomoto and H. Masuda, A study of pyrazine formation, *J. Agric. Food Chem.*, **27**, 1027–31 (1979).

53. A. Ferretti, V. P. Flanagan and J. M. Ruth, Nonenzymatic browning in a lactose-casein model system, *J. Agric. Food Chem.*, **18**, 13–18 (1970).

54. G. Vernin and G. Vernin, Heterocyclic aroma compounds in foods: occurrence and organoleptic properties, in *The Chemistry of Heterocyclic Flavoring and Aroma Compounds* (ed. G. Vernin), Ellis Horwood Publishers, Chichester, pp. 72–150.

55. J. E. Hodge, Origin of flavor in foods — nonenzymatic browning reactions, in *Symposium on Foods, Chemistry and Physiology of Flavors* (eds. H. W. Schultz, E. A. Day and L. M. Libbey), The AVI Publishing Co., Westport, Connecticut, 1967, pp. 465–91.

56. O. G. Vitzthum, P. Werkhoff and P. J. Hubert, Volatile components of roasted cocoa: basic fraction, *J. Food Sci.*, **408**, 911–14 (1975).

57. J. Stoffelsma, G. Sipma, D. K. Kettenes and J. Pypker, New volatile components of roasted coffee, *J. Agric. Food Chem.*, **16**, 1000–4 (1968).

58. S. S. Chang and R. J. Peterson, Symposium: the basis of quality in muscle foods: recent developments in flavor of meat, *J. Food Sci.*, **42**, 298–305 (1977).

59. R. J. Harding, J. J. Wren and H. E. Nursten, Volatile basic compounds derived from roasted barley, *J. Inst. Brew.*, **84**, 41–2 (1978).

60. E. C. Coleman, C.-T. Ho and S. S. Chang, Isolation and identification of volatile compounds from baked potatoes, *J. Agric. Food Chem.*, **29**, 42–8 (1981).

61. M. H. Lee, C.-T. Ho and S. S. Chang, Thiazoles, oxazoles and oxazolines identified in the volatile flavor of roasted peanuts, *J. Agric. Food Chem.*, **29**, 684–6 (1981).

62. C.-T. Ho, Q. Z. Jin, K. N. Lee, J. T. Carlin and S. S. Chang, Synthesis and aroma properties of new alkyloxazoles and alkylthiazoles identified in cocoa butter from roasted cocoa beans, *J. Food Sci.*, **48**, 1570–1 (1983).

63. J. T. Carlin, Q. Z. Jin, T. Z. Huang, C.-T. Ho and S. S. Chang, Identification of alkyloxazoles in the volatile compounds from french fried potatoes, *J. Agric. Food Chem.*, **34**, 621–3 (1986).

64. S. S. Chang, C. Hirai, B. R. Reddy, K. O. Herz and G. Sigma, Isolation and identification of 2,4,5-trimethyl-3-oxazoline and 2,5-dimethyl-1,2,4-trithiolane in the volatile flavor compounds of boiled beef, *Chem. Ind. (Lond.)*, 1639 (1968).

65. C. J. Mussinan, R. A. Wilson, I. Katz, A. Hruza and M. H. Vock, Identification and flavor properties of some 3-oxazolines and 3-thiazolines isolated from cooked beef, in *Phenolic, Sulfur, and Nitrogen Compounds in Food Flavors* (eds. G. Charalambous and I. Katz), ACS Symposium Series 26, American Chemical Society, Washington, D.C., 1976, pp. 133–45.

66. R. J. Peterson, H. J. Izzo, E. Jungermann and S. S. Chang, Changes in volatile flavor compounds during the retorting of canned beef stew, *J. Food Sci.*, **40**, 948–54 (1975).

67. C.-T. Ho and G. J. Hartman, Formation of oxazolines and oxazoles in Strecker degradation of DL-alanine and L-cysteine with 2,3-butanedione, *J. Agric. Food Chem.*, **30**, 793–4 (1982).

68. L. J. Farmer and D. S. Mottram, Lipid–Maillard interactions in the formation of volatile aroma compounds, in *Trends in Flavour Research* (eds. H. Maarse and D. G. van der Heij), Elsevier Science B. V., Amsterdam, 1994, pp. 313–26.

69. F. B. Whitefield, Volatiles from interactions of Maillard reactions and lipids, *Crit. Rev. Food Sci. Nutr.*, **31**, 1–58 (1992).

70. E. M. Chiu, M. C. Kuo, L. J. Bruechert and C.-T. Ho, Substitution of pyrazines by aldehydes in model systems, *J. Agric. Food Chem.*, **38**, 58–61 (1990).

71. J. Tang, Q. Z. Jin, G. H. Shen, C.-T. Ho and S. S. Chang, isolation and identification of volatile compounds in fried chicken, *J. Agric. Food Chem.*, **31**, 1287–92 (1983).

72. C.-T. Ho and J. T. Carlin, Formation and aroma characteristics of heterocyclic compounds in foods, in *Flavor Chemistry: Trends and Developments* (eds. R. Teranishi, R. G. Buttery and F. Shahidi), ACS Symposium Series 388, American Chemical Society, Washington, D.C. 1989, pp. 92–104.

73. M. Stoll, P. Dietrich, E. Sundte and M. Winter, Recherches sur les arômes. Sur l'arôme de cocao, II, *Helv. Chim. Acta*, **50**, 2065–7 (1967).

74. H. J. Takken, L. M. van der Linde, P. J. de Valois, J. M. van Dort and M. Boelens, Reaction products of α-dicarbonyl compounds, aldehydes, hydrogen sulfide, and ammonia, in *Phenolic, Sulfur, and Nitrogen Compounds in Food Flavors* (eds. G. Charalambous and I. Katz), ACS Symposium Series 26, American Chemical Society, Washington, D.C., 1976, pp. 114–21.

75. G. R. Rizzi, A. R. Steimle and D. R. Patton, Formation of dialkylthiophenes in Maillard reactions involving cysteine, in *Food Science and Nutrition* (ed. G. Charalambous), Elsevier Science Publishers B. V., Amsterdam, 1992, pp. 731–41.

3

The Role of Oxidation in the Maillard Reaction *in vivo**

JOHN W. BAYNES

Department of Chemistry and Biochemistry and School of Medicine,
University of South Carolina, USA

INTRODUCTION—THE MAILLARD REACTION IN FOOD CHEMISTRY AND BIOLOGICAL SYSTEMS

The chemistry of the Maillard reaction in food products[1,2] includes a range of reactions of unsaturated lipids and reducing sugars with amino, sulfhydryl, guanidino and other functional groups in biomolecules. A common feature of the most reactive lipids and carbohydrates is their susceptibility to oxidation. The term 'reducing sugar' is indeed a chemical affirmation of the ease of oxidation of dietary monosaccharides (glucose, fructose) and disaccharides (lactose, maltose), and food chemists have long recognized that control of the Maillard reaction requires control of the oxidation chemistry of lipids and carbohydrates. To inhibit oxidation chemistry and prevent the deterioration in appearance and nutritional value of foods, they are commonly stored at low relative humidity, hermetically sealed under vacuum or anaerobic conditions, and fortified with antioxidants, such as butylated hydroxytoluene and bisulfite. Chelators are also added to processed foods to inhibit catalysis of both carbohydrate and lipid oxidation reactions by traces of transition metal ions, particularly iron and copper. Ene-diol structures are intermediates in metal-catalyzed oxidation of carbohydrates, and shorter chain sugars, which enolize more rapidly than hexoses, oxidize more readily than hexoses.[3] Ascorbate, a naturally occurring ene-diol, is often used as a sacrificial antioxidant in foods. It is not only more easily oxidized than other sugars, but, as a reducing agent,

---

*Dedicated to the memory of Dr Simon P. Wolff, a pioneer in research on autoxidative glycosylation and the role of oxidation in the Maillard reaction *in vivo*.

The Maillard Reaction: Consequences for the Chemical and Life Sciences. Edited by Raphael Ikan
©1996 John Wiley & Sons Ltd

inhibits browning reactions by reducing catalytic metal ions and reactive carbohydrate intermediates in oxidation reactions. Lipids also vary widely in their susceptibility to oxidation, polyunsaturated fatty acids in lipids being more readily oxidized than either unsaturated or monounsaturated fatty acids. Initiation of the oxidation of either carbohydrates or lipids stimulates the oxidation of the other, and these autoxidation reactions generate reactive oxygen species, including peroxides, oxygen radicals and metal–oxo complexes. Reactive carbonyl intermediates are also formed in these reactions, including dicarbonyl sugars from carbohydrates and aldehydes and their derivatives from lipids, which are directly involved in the browning and crosslinking reactions characteristic of the Maillard reaction.

Only in the last 10–15 years have biomedical scientists begun to appreciate the significance of nonenzymatic, Maillard, reactions *in vivo* and their relevance to chemical modification of proteins and other biomolecules during natural aging and in diseases such as diabetes and atherosclerosis.[4,5] A generalized enhancement of nonenzymatic oxidation chemistry, known as 'oxidative stress', is also implicated in the pathogenesis of these and other diseases,[6] and the interplay between the Maillard reaction and oxidative stress has become a fruitful area for study. Evidence is now accumulating which indicates that oxidation chemistry modulates the impact of the Maillard reaction *in vivo*.[7,8] Reactive oxygen species are formed in metabolic reactions, particularly as side products of mitochondrial electron transport, and also in nonenzymatic autoxidation reactions involving oxidizable substrates, metal ions and molecular oxygen. Although DNA and protein may be damaged directly in oxidation reactions, the carbonyl products formed on oxidation of carbohydrates and lipids also react with these targets, further extending the damage. In addition, the nonoxidative adduction of sugars to proteins or nucleic acids yields Schiff bases and Amadori adducts which enhance the generation of reactive oxygen by reducing sugars. Much of the damage resulting from these oxidation reactions is corrected by repair and turnover processes. Proteins, however, are not repairable, and the resultant intra- and intermolecular crosslinking can affect their structure, recognition and function. This is particularly true for long-lived proteins, such as collagens and lens crystallins, which have half-lives measured in years in human tissues and therefore accumulate modifications over significant periods of time.

As described below, carbohydrates contribute to the chemical modification and crosslinking of collagen during aging, and these reactions are thought to contribute, in turn, to the altered elasticity of collagen, decreased compliance of the vascular wall and changes in permeability of renal and vascular basement membranes with age. Modification of proteins by carbohydrates is accelerated during hyperglycemia in diabetes and is implicated in the development of the long-term complications of this disease, including retinopathy, nephropathy and generalized vascular disease.[7,8] The characteristic carbohydrate-derived products which accumulate in tissue proteins with age and at an accelerated rate in diabetes are products of both glycation and oxidation reactions, emphasizing the interplay between glycation and oxidation chemistry. This overview will focus on the significance of reactions between carbohydrates and proteins in aging and disease and on the importance of oxidation reactions as catalysts of chemical modification of proteins via the Maillard reactions *in vivo*.

ROLE OF OXYGEN AS A CATALYST OF THE MAILLARD REACTION

Much of the early research on the Maillard reaction[1,2] was focused on its role in development and deterioration of flavor, taste and nutritional value of foods during processing and storage. The chemistry was often carried out at nonphysiological conditions, at extremes of temperature and pH, or in organic solvents. In 1953, in his comprehensive review of Maillard reactions of carbohydrates, Hodge[1] identified the Schiff base as a precursor and the Amadori compound as the first stable product, formed on reaction of reducing sugars with protein. He also identified deoxyosones, furfurals, reductones (easily oxidized ene-diol sugar derivatives), and low molecular weight carbonyl and dicarbonyl fission products as intermediates formed in the second stage of the reaction, leading eventually to the formation of brown, insoluble pigments, known as melanoidins, in the third or final stage. Ledl and Schleicher[9] more recently reviewed the evidence for involvement of dicarbonyl sugars, 1-, 3- and 4-deoxyaldosuloses, as intermediates in the Maillard reaction. These deoxy-osones may be formed directly from the reducing sugars, but the reaction is catalyzed by amines via Amadori compounds (Figure 3.1, left side). Feather[10] noted that the relative rates of formation of the various deoxyglucosones from Amadori compounds depended on the pH of the medium, with acidic pH favoring 1-deoxyglucosone formation and alkaline pH favoring 3-deoxyglu-cosone. In all these pathways, the deoxyglucosones are products of rearrangement and dehydration reactions; thus there are well-characterized pathways to the formation of dicarbonyl sugar intermediates in the Maillard reaction without invoking a requirement for oxidation chemistry.

In 1987, Kato *et al.*[11] identified 3-deoxyglucosone as an intermediate in the browning of protein by glucose in physiological buffers. Szwergold *et al.*[12] also showed that 3-deoxyglucosone could be formed by elimination of phosphate from fructose-3-phosphate (Figure 3.1, center), while 1-deoxyglucosone could be formed in the same fashion from fructose-1-phosphate. Wells-Knecht *et al.*[13] and Niwa *et al.*[14] subsequently identified 3-deoxyglucosone in human plasma, supporting its role as a Maillard reaction intermediate *in vivo*. Glomb *et al.*[15] have also presented evidence for formation of 1-deoxyglucosone during reaction of glucose with protein under physiological conditions and Ledl and

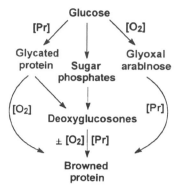

Figure 3.1. Role of dicarbonyl intermediates in oxidative and nonoxidative pathways of the Maillard reactions. (Left) Nonoxidative pathway leading to the formation of Amadori adducts which rearrange and hydrolyze to form deoxyglucosones which[9,10] which brown protein under either oxidative or antioxidative conditions. (Centre) Nonoxidative pathway involving sugar phosphates as a source of deoxyglucosones.[11] (Right) Autoxidative glycosylation pathway leading to the formation of glyoxal and arabinose;[21,25] glyoxal and arabinose are precursors to glycoxidation products, CML and P, respectively. The various pathways converge on dicarbonyl sugars, which mediate the browning and crosslinking of proteins

Schleicher[9] for formation of 4-deoxyglucosone or its derivatives. However, with the exception of 3-deoxyglucosone, these compounds have been detected only in model reaction systems by trapping them as derivatives of dicarbonyl reagents, such as aminoguanidine or *o*-phenylenediamine. Konishi *et al.*[16] have characterized imidazolone adducts formed by reaction of 3-deoxyglucosone with the guanidino group of arginine derivatives and Lo *et al.*[17] have described similar products in reactions of methylglyoxal with albumin *in vitro*. Although these imidazolone adducts, or other products derived uniquely from deoxyglucosones, have not been detected in biological systems, the general role of dicarbonyl sugars in browning reactions is supported, not only by the work of Kato *et al.*,[11] but also by studies of Ortwerth *et al.*[18] and Dunn *et al.*,[19] showing that the browning of protein by ascorbate first requires the oxidation of ascorbate to the dicarbonyl sugar, dehydroascorbate. Browning of proteins by dehydroascorbate, as well as deoxyosones, then proceeds under anaerobic conditions. Simpler dicarbonyl sugars, such as glyoxal and methylglyoxal, also brown proteins rapidly in the absence of oxygen.

Although Maillard reactions proceed under anaerobic conditions, the rate of browning of protein by hexoses is slow in the absence of air. Based on the kinetics of browning reactions involving glucose, Hayashi and Namiki[20] concluded that both oxidation reactions and free radical intermediates were involved at the earliest stages of this reaction. They proposed that fragmentation of Schiff base adducts, prior to the Amadori rearrangement, led to the formation of 2- and 3-carbon dicarbonyl sugars, which then proceeded to form melanoidins. Wolff and Dean[21] also observed that the rate of reaction of glucose with protein was greatly accelerated in the presence of oxygen and transition metals, leading to the development of their *autoxidative glycosylation* hypothesis.[7] According to this hypothesis (Figure 3.1, right side), metal-catalyzed autoxidation (oxidation by molecular oxygen) of glucose itself is the rate-limiting step in the chemical modification of proteins by glucose. Chase *et al.*[22] and Fu *et al.*[23,24] later showed that the crosslinking and browning of collagen by glucose was, in fact, critically dependent on autoxidative conditions, i.e. the presence of molecular oxygen with transition metal ion catalysts, although the substrate for the autoxidation reaction, e.g. glucose, the Schiff base or Amadori adduct, was not identified. Using Girard-T reagent, Wolff and Dean[21] had originally shown that dicarbonyl sugars were formed during autoxidative glycosylation by glucose, and Wells-Knecht *et al.*[25] recently identified arabinose and the dicarbonyl compound, glyoxal, as products of autoxidation of glucose in phosphate buffer under physiological conditions. 3-Aminotriazine, the product of the reaction between glyoxal and aminoguanidine, has now been identified as a major product formed during inhibition of the browning of collagen by glucose under oxidative conditions (K. J. Wells-Knecht, personal communication). From this same reaction mixture, Blackledge *et al.*[26] isolated two 3-carbon adducts to aminoguanidine, suggesting that glucose decomposed to form triose reductone, which was a precursor to glyoxal.

The overall conclusion from these studies is that dicarbonyl sugars are involved in both nonoxidative and autoxidative pathways of the Maillard reaction, i.e. deoxyglucosones under antioxidative conditions and glyoxal under oxidative conditions (Figure 3.1). The importance of oxidation chemistry in the Maillard reaction depends on the carbohydrate. For ascorbate, oxidation appears to be essential;[18] for glucose, oxidation is rate limiting;[21–24] and for pentoses and tetroses, the rates of browning and crosslinking of proteins are comparable in the presence and absence of oxygen (J. E. Litchfield, personal communication). Glyoxal has been identified as the common dicarbonyl intermediate formed on autoxidation of glucose, fructose and arabinose under oxidative conditions, and the greater rate of browning of proteins by fructose, compared to glucose, can be attributed to the more rapid oxidation and formation of glyoxal from fructose. Other reactive dicarbonyls, such as methylglyoxal (pyruvaldehyde)[17,27] or triose reductone[1,2] formed either enzymatically or nonenzymatically, may also contribute to the Maillard reaction *in vivo*.

ADVANCED GLYCATION END-PRODUCTS (AGEs)

Cerami and colleagues[28] introduced the term, AGE, an acronym for advanced glycosylation (now glycation) end-product, to describe the brown, fluorescent and crosslinking compounds that accumulate in tissue proteins with age. The initial characterization of AGEs as carbohydrate-derived compounds was based on the similarity in brown color and fluorescence which accumulate with age in natural proteins, e.g. lens crystallins and tissue collagens, and the physical and structural changes occurring during Maillard reactions between sugars and proteins *in vitro*. The term, AGE, is a useful play on words, since AGEs accumulate in long-lived proteins with chronological *age*. Like the structure of melanoidins, the structures of the majority of AGEs are unknown. However, artificial AGEs or AGE-proteins may be prepared *in vitro* by incubating a protein for 1–3 months in concentrated glucose solution in 0.2–0.5 M phosphate buffer at neutral pH. The physiological relevance of AGEs is confirmed by the observations that antibodies prepared against AGE-proteins react with antigens in tissue proteins,[29] that these AGE antigens increase in human lens proteins with age[30] and that they are present at higher age-adjusted levels in human serum[31] and red cell[32] proteins in diabetes, and in aortic[31] and renal[33] collagen in diabetic rats. AGE proteins and peptides are also found in plasma where their concentrations increase in diabetic patients receiving hemodialysis therapy for end-stage renal disease,[31] implicating the kidney in the clearance and/or catabolism of AGEs on circulating proteins. Recently, Bucala *et al.*[34] also measured AGEs on low-density lipoprotein (LDL) and showed that AGE-LDL increased in hemodialysis patients, independent of diabetes, further supporting the role of the kidney in the removal of circulating AGE-proteins.

The meaning of the term, AGE, has evolved over time, and AGE is now used as a general descriptor for nearly any protein-bound product formed during the advanced or browning stages of the Maillard reaction (Figure 3.2), including, for example, N^ε-(carboxymethyl)lysine (CML),[35] N^ε-(3-lactato)lysine[36] and pyrraline,[37] which are nether fluorescent nor crosslinks, nor is there evidence that the latter two compounds accumulate in proteins with age. Thus far, only three structurally characterized AGEs have been documented to accumulate with age in tissue proteins: CML,[35] the analogous carboxymethyl derivative of hydroxylysine, N^ε-(carboxymethyl)hydroxylysine (CMhL)[38] and pentosidine.[35,39] Among them, only pentosidine is a fluorescent crosslink, bridging an arginine and a lysine residue in protein(s). CML and pentosidine are detectable at low levels in plasma proteins,[40] but accumulate to higher levels with age in long-lived proteins, such as lens proteins and tissue collagens.[35,38,39] CML, pentosidine and Maillard-type fluorescence are also present at higher age-adjusted levels in skin collagen from diabetic patients, particularly those with complications.[41–45] Increased levels of pentosidine have also been detected in plasma proteins and peptides of persons with diabetes and/or end-stage renal disease,[40] and increased levels of CML have been detected in the urine of diabetic patients.[46] In studies in model systems, Nakamura *et al.*[47] have recently characterized an epimeric pair of glucose-derived fluorescent, lysine–lysine crosslinks, termed 'crosslines', and reported increased levels of immunoreactive crosslines in kidney proteins of diabetic rats. However, age-dependent accumulation of crosslines has not been demonstrated, nor have they been isolated from tissue proteins. Overall, although there is wide variation in physical, chemical and biological properties among compounds currently recognized as AGEs (Figure 3.2), they share in common their formation during later stages of the Maillard reaction.

GLYCOXIDATION PRODUCTS

Fu *et al.*[23,24] observed that autoxidative conditions, i.e. traces of transition metal catalysts and molecular oxygen, were required for the formation of the AGEs, CML and pentosidine (Figure 3.2) during the browning and crosslinking of collagen by glucose. The term 'glycoxidation product' was introduced to describe these compounds, as well as N^{ε}-(3-lactato) lysine[36] and CMhL,[38] all of which required both glycation and oxidation reactions for their formation from glucose. The glycoxidation products, CML and pentosidine, not only accumulate with age in proteins *in vivo* but also accumulate at an accelerated rate as a result of hyperglycemia and increased glycation of protein in diabetes. Lyons *et al.*[48] showed that, during a four-month period of improved glycemic control in diabetic patients (documented by decreases in mean blood glucose and glycated hemoglobin), glycation of skin collagen decreased significantly, whereas CML, CMhL, pentosidine and fluorescence in collagen remained unchanged. Based on these observations, oxygen, via autoxidation or glycoxidation reactions, was judged to be a fixative of Maillard reaction damage to proteins, yielding irreversible chemical damage, equivalent to the rusting of proteins.[8,48,49]

In contrast to autoxidative glycosylation, in which autoxidation of sugars is followed by glycation of protein[7,21] or to the Namiki pathway[20] in which reaction of sugar with protein is followed by oxidation reactions, glycoxidation is considered to result from the net effects of glycation and oxidation reactions, in either order. Indeed, it is difficult to determine which comes first, glycation or oxidation. Because of the low equilibrium constant of the reaction, the concentration of Amadori adducts on protein is always lower than the ambient glucose concentration. However, Amadori adducts are more readily oxidized than glucose, and, in fact, selective oxidation of Amadori compounds in the presence of free glucose is the basis for the fructosamine assay for glycated proteins.[50] Thus, even though Amadori compounds are present at lower concentrations than glucose in blood (estimated 0.5–1 mM concentration of Amadori adducts on plasma proteins,[51] compared to 5 mM free glucose), the Amadori adducts, being more easily oxidized, may contribute significantly to the formation of glycoxidation products. In studies *in vitro*, Chace *et al.*[22] concluded that oxidation of glucose preceded the crosslinking and browning of

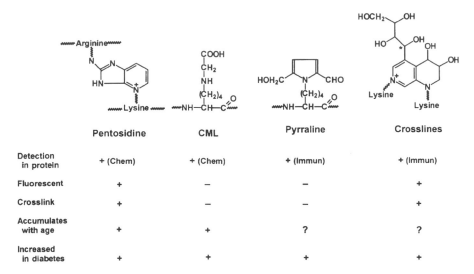

	Pentosidine	CML	Pyrraline	Crosslines
Detection in protein	+ (Chem)	+ (Chem)	+ (Immun)	+ (Immun)
Fluorescent	+	−	−	+
Crosslink	+	−	−	+
Accumulates with age	+	+	?	?
Increased in diabetes	+	+	+	+

Figure 3.2. The structures and properties of advanced glycosylation end-products (AGEs) which have been detected in proteins *in vivo*

collagen by glucose, i.e. in support of autoxidative glycosylation, while Hunt *et al.*[52] demonstrated that glycation of albumin preceded oxidation and cleavage of the protein by glucose, challenging the autoxidative glycosylation hypothesis. In our laboratory, when collagen was pre-glycated under antioxidative conditions with natural glucose, then incubated with [U–^{13}C]-glucose under oxidative conditions, the yields of ^{12}C– and ^{13}C–CML were used to estimate the relative rates of oxidation of both Amadori products and free glucose to form CML. We observed that oxidation of both Amadori adducts and glucose proceeded simultaneously during glycoxidation reactions *in vitro*.[53] However, the relative rates of oxidation of Amadori adducts and glucose varied up to tenfold with changes in glucose, phosphate and metal ion concentrations (M. C. Wells-Knecht, personal communication). Thus, the concentrations and species of metal ions and buffers affect not only the kinetics of glycoxidation reactions *in vitro* but also the relative rates of oxidation of Amadori adducts and glucose. There is some debate about the physiological relevance of these studies *in vitro* because it is unlikely that similar concentrations of free transition metal ions would be attained *in vivo*.[54] However, oxidation reactions may be catalyzed in microenvironments abnormally rich in decompartmentalized metal ions, e.g. at sites of inflammation, or by metal–protein complexes.[55] It is likely that metal ion-*in*dependent oxidation reactions, mediated by hydroperoxy radicals (the protonated, more reactive form of superoxide), hypochlorous acid or peroxynitrite, may also contribute to formation of glycoxidation products and AGEs *in vivo*. In summary, since both free carbohydrates and their adducts to protein are subject to autoxidation, glycation and oxidation reactions probably proceed in either sequence toward the formation of glycoxidation products *in vivo*. Numerous sugars may also contribute to the formation of the same glycoxidation product, e.g. CML may be formed from hexoses, ascorbate, pentoses, tetroses and glyoxal,[19,20,25] while pentosidine, which contains five carbohydrate-derived carbons, may be formed from hexoses, pentoses, ascorbate and even tetroses.[56,57] At this time, because only a limited number of end-products of Maillard reactions between sugars and proteins have been characterized, and none of these are unique to any one sugar, it is not yet possible to determine the relative contribution of various sugars to the browning of protein *in vivo*.

Regardless of the reaction sequence or carbohydrate precursor, levels of glycoxidation products are closely correlated with the browning and cross-linking of collagen by glucose *in vitro*, and, as noted above, age-adjusted levels of CML and pentosidine are disproportionately increased in skin collagen from diabetic patients with complications.[42–45] Because of the possible involvement of glycoxidation in the pathogenesis of diabetic complications, pharmacological inhibition of the Maillard reaction is a logical target for therapeutic intervention. A number of compounds have now been described which inhibit the formation of glycoxidation products *in vitro*, simultaneous with inhibition of the browning and crosslinking of collagen by glucose. These inhibitors include a range of compounds with antioxidant activity, including chelators (diethylenetriaminepentaacetic acid, phytic acid, penicillamine), reducing agents (dithiothreitol, glutathione, penicillamine, lipoic acid) and radical scavengers (thiourea, tiron, aspirin, salicylate),[24,58] as well as aminoguanidine, which is not an antioxidant but traps reactive dicarbonyl sugar intermediates formed during Maillard reactions under either antioxidative or autoxidative conditions. Studies in animal models of diabetes (reviewed in Ref. 8) indicate that treatment with antioxidant or anti-inflammatory drugs, such as penicillamine (both a reducing agent and a chelator) and nonsteroidal anti-inflammatory drugs (including aspirin, salicylate and lipoxygenase inhibitors), also inhibits the development of chemical and physical changes in collagen and alterations in the vascular permeability characteristic of diabetes. Similar effects are observed with aldose reductase inhibitors, which correct tissue redox imbalances resulting from excessive polyol pathway activity in diabetes (reviewed in Refs. 8 and 59). Although the protective effects of these drugs are consistent with a role for glycoxidation in development of diabetic complications, the drugs may also cause a generalized decrease in inflammation and/or oxidative stress, affecting prostanoid metabolism and nonenzymatic lipid peroxidation, so that their effects are not limited to inhibition of glycoxidation alone. Similarly, aminoguanidine inhibits the accelerated browning and crosslinking of collagen in diabetic animals and delays or prevents the appearance of long-term diabetic complications, including nephropathy, retinopathy, neuropathy and vascular disease (reviewed in Ref. 59). However, the mechanism of therapeutic action of aminoguanidine is still uncertain since it can trap dicarbonyl sugars formed in both nonoxidative and autoxidative pathways of the Maillard reaction of carbohydrates or trap reactive aldehydes formed during oxidation of lipids in lipoproteins,[60] but it also inhibits the activity of enzymes such as amine oxidase and nitric oxide synthetase, which may affect vascular and neural processes. In summary, the therapeutic effects of antioxidants, anti-inflammatory agents and amino-guanidine are consistent with, but do not establish unequivocally, the role of glycoxidation reactions in the development of diabetic complications.

Although the results of pharmacological intervention are inconclusive, there is some evidence from clinical studies that glycoxidation may be the critical factor in the development of long-term complications of diabetes.[61–63] Dyer et al.[35] noted that, in general, the increase in age-corrected levels of glycoxidation products in skin collagen from diabetic patients could be explained by their age, duration of diabetes and the mean increase in glycemia,[35] estimated from the extent of glycation of collagen. Thus, it was not necessary to invoke an increase in oxidative stress as a general feature of the diabetic state. However, although the number of patients was limited and the conclusion only marginally significant ($0.1 > p > 0.05$), patients with higher age-corrected levels of glycoxidation products, but comparable glycemic control, appeared to be at greater risk for development of complications.[44] These correlations suggest that 'glycoxidative stress',[61–63] the mathematical product of glycative and oxidative stress, is increased in the subpopulation of diabetic patients with more severe complications. From this perspective, oxidative stress may be viewed as a modulator of the rate of the Maillard reaction and the consequences of hyperglycemia in diabetes. Patients with similar duration of diabetes and severity of glycemia, but with higher 'set points' for oxidative stress because of genetic or nutritional effects on antioxidant defences, may therefore be more susceptible to complications. Thus, both control of glycemia (glycative stress) and reduction in oxidative stress should have beneficial effects in the treatment of diabetes. Williamson et al[64] have also proposed that hyperglycemia induces a chronic state of 'pseudohypoxia' in tissues, a condition with metabolic similarities to ischemia and characterized by increased oxidative stress resulting from altered cellular redox potentials. According to this hypothesis, correction of hyperglycemia would decrease both glycative and oxidative stress simultaneously. It is noteworthy that diabetic patients, in addition to receiving instruction in the maintenance of good glycemic control, are generally treated in a holistic manner which leads simultaneously to a decrease in oxidative stress, independent of any decrease in glycemia. Thus, the encouragement to stop smoking, an independent risk factor for vascular disease, would yield a decrease in oxidative stress and theoretically reduce the risk of complications. Similarly, a balanced diet, rich in fruits and vegetables, would provide enhanced vitamin-dependent antioxidant defences, possibly also contributing to a decreased risk for development of complications in diabetes. At this time, the role of autoxidation and oxidative stress in catalysis of the Maillard reaction *in vivo* and the significance of glycoxidative stress in the development of diabetic complications are still hypothetical. The resolution of these issues will depend on the development of reliable indices of endogenous oxidative stress, clinical assessment of the effects of antioxidant therapy and a more complete understanding of the mechanism of action of various drugs, including antioxidants, aldose reductase inhibitors and aminoguanidine, which retard the development of diabetic complications in animals or humans.

In addition to their relevance to diabetes, the formation and accumulation of glycoxidation products in tissue proteins provides a direct link between the Maillard reaction and the free radical theory of aging. This theory proposes that aging is the result of chronic chemical damage to biomolecules by oxygen radical chemistry. Since oxygen radicals are involved in the formation of glycoxidation products, the age-dependent accumulation of glycoxidation products in tissue protein constitutes evidence in support of the free radical theory. Monnier has proposed a Maillard theory of aging[65] which encompasses both oxidative and nonoxidative modifications of protein with age. However, the only identified Maillard products known to accumulate with age in proteins are the glycoxidation products,[8] which involve oxygen radical chemistry in their formation. Thus the Maillard theory of aging may be seen as one aspect of the free radical theory. Diabetes, a disease in which the accumulation of glycoxidation products is accelerated, may then be viewed as a disease of accelerated aging of tissue proteins and other biomolecules. This accelerated aging, coupled with the metabolic derangements of diabetes, may contribute to the development of diabetic complications. Recent work suggests that AGEs may also accelerate the deposition of amyloid plaque in hemodialysis-associated amyloidosis[66] and of β-amyloid protein in the brain in Alzheimer's disease.[67]

RELATIONSHIP BETWEEN AGEs AND GLYCOXIDATION PRODUCTS

Anti-AGE antibodies have proven to be useful immunochemical reagents for assessing the extent of chemical modification of tissue proteins by Maillard reactions. In the preparation of the AGE-proteins used as immunogens, antioxidative conditions have not been rigorously maintained, so that, in fact, AGE-proteins contain glycoxidation products. Indeed, in AGE-proteins prepared by published procedures,[31,68,69] we find that considerable glycoxidation has occurred, yielding 20–30% conversion of lysine residues to CML in AGE-protein preparations. However, even if glycoxidation products were not present in the original AGE-protein immunogen, they might be formed on the protein *in situ* as a result of inflammation and oxidative stress at the site of immunization, particularly when adjuvants are used to stimulate the immune response. In ELISA assays using two separate polyclonal antibodies prepared in our laboratory against AGE-proteins, we have observed that a range of sugars, including glucose, fructose, arabinose and even glyoxal, produce AGEs during incubation with model proteins and low molecular weight lysine derivatives. The formation of AGEs from glucose and fructose in these model systems was essentially completely inhibited under antioxidative conditions. Thus the AGEs recognized by our anti-AGE antibodies appeared to be glycoxidation products.

Confirming previous work by Horiuchi *et al.*[68] and Nakayama *et al.*,[69] we have shown that a common AGE structure is formed from various sugars, including glucose, fructose, ascorbate, arabinose and glyoxal, and have recently identified CML as a dominant immunological determinant on AGE proteins.[70] The requirement for oxygen in the formation of AGE protein from glucose and fructose is consistent with the fact that autoxidative conditions are required for the formation of CML from these sugars, while glyoxal, which forms AGEs under both oxidative and antioxidative conditions, also yields CML at comparable rates under oxidative and antioxidative conditions.[25] Although Makita *et al.*[31] have previously reported that anti-AGE antibodies do not recognize any of the known determinants in browned proteins, including CML, pentosidine and pyrraline, we have observed that free CML and N^{α}-(acetyl)CML are $\leqslant 0.1\%$ as effective as CML-containing peptides as competitors in ELISA assays for AGEs. This observation explains the apparent destruction of AGEs on acid hydrolysis of proteins, and is consistent with reports that AGEs are not reducible by $NaBH_4$. Indeed, we have found, with both of our antibodies, that chemically carboxymethylated proteins completely inhibited the recognition of AGEs in artificial AGE proteins and in human lens proteins in a competitive ELISA assay, suggesting that CML (or closely related compounds) is the major determinant recognized in ELISA assays for AGEs in tissue proteins.[70] Our results also suggest that the recognition of AGE proteins by the scavenger receptor,[71] which has specificity for polyanionic compounds,[72] may be explained by the presence of CML residues on the surface on the AGE protein. Since it is a major determinant on AGE proteins, CML could also be the recognition element for the AGE–receptor (RAGE) complex.[73] Other AGEs are undoubtedly present on AGE proteins, but, in addition to being poorly characterized, may be weakly immunogenic, perhaps because of their structural heterogeneity and thus the low concentration of individual species in the AGE protein immunogens. Our observations suggest that monoclonal antibodies which do not cross-react with CML will be more useful than polyclonal antibodies for the detection, immunoaffinity isolation and structural characterization of new AGEs and/or glycoxidation products in tissue proteins. The significance of oxidation in the Maillard reaction *in vivo* would be confirmed if other AGEs detected in tissue proteins were also identified as glycoxidation products.

INTERPLAY BETWEEN GLYCOXIDATION AND OXIDATION IN LIPOPROTEINS

The oxidation of glucose, Schiff bases, Amadori adducts and more reactive intermediates during glycoxidation reactions generates reactive oxygen species, which then produce *o*-tyrosine and methionine sulfoxide in protein (M. C. Wells-Knecht, personal communication) and lead to fragmentation and crosslinking of proteins.[55] Glycation of lipoproteins also promotes lipid peroxidation reactions,[74] leading to speculation that glycation and glycoxidation may accelerate oxidative modification of lipoproteins in diabetes, promoting the development of vascular disease.[75] However, despite evidence that low-density lipoprotein (LDL) isolated from diabetic patients is more susceptible to oxidation *in vitro* and that susceptibility to oxidation correlates with the extent of glycation of the protein,[76] there is no published evidence that LDL glycation is correlated with LDL lipid peroxidation or vascular disease in diabetes.[77] Bucala *et al.*[78] have reported recently that levels of AGEs are increased on LDL isolated from serum of diabetic patients and that glycation of LDL *in vitro* promotes both the formation of AGEs and the peroxidation of LDL lipids. Glycation of LDL was not measured in these experiments, but there were significant correlations between the AGE and lipid peroxide content of the LDL, measured by the thiobarbituric acid reaction as malondialdehyde equivalents. Although the status of vascular disease in the patients was not reported, these studies suggest that AGE–LDL, rather than glycated LDL, may be the more relevant species involved in the pathogenesis of diabetic vascular disease. It is interesting to note that AGE–LDL is also increased, independent of an increase in glycation, in nondiabetic patients with end-stage renal disease.[78] These patients are at high risk for the development of vascular disease, consistent with a role for AGEing, rather than glycation, of LDL in the development of vascular disease. The two processes, glycation and AGEing, may be dissociated, especially for LDL, since the rate of conversion of glycated LDL to AGE–LDL and subsequent damage from lipid peroxidation reactions may depend on numerous factors, including the inherent oxidizability of LDL lipids, the LDL content of antioxidant vitamins and the individual's overall status of oxidative stress. Clarifying the relationship between glycation and AGEing of LDL in diabetic and nondiabetic vascular disease will be essential for understanding the role of glycation, AGEing and lipoprotein oxidation in the development of vascular disease.

Bucala *et al.*[34] also reported that lipoprotein glycation was not confined to the protein component of LDL, but that lipids, such as phosphatidylethanolamine, were also modified in LDL to form AGEs, adding another level of complexity to the Maillard reaction *in vivo*. We have, in fact, recently detected fructose–ethanol-amine, the Amadori adduct of glucose to ethanolamine, in human urine, supporting the argument that phosphatidylethanolamine (and probably phosphatidylserine) is glycated *in vivo*. We speculate that the AGE–phosphatidyl-ethanolamine structure in LDL may be *N*-(carboxymethyl)-phosphatidylethanolamine. This compound, the glycoxidation product of glycated phosphatidylethanolamine, may share sufficient structural homology with CML (Figure 3.2) to cross-react in the AGE ELISA assay. Bucala *et al.*[34] have also shown that AGE peptides, which are elevated in the serum of patients with diabetes or end-stage renal disease, react with LDL to yield an increase in AGEs in both the protein and lipid components of LDL. AGEing of LDL inhibited recognition and catabolism of LDL by the apo-B,E receptor, leading to the proposal that formation of AGEs on LDL may contribute to elevated levels of LDL and dyslipidemia in patients with diabetes or renal impairment. It is not clear, however, why AGE–LDL is not cleared by the AGE[79] or RAGE[73] receptors which are widely distributed in tissues.[80] Perhaps the level of AGEs (or CML) is sufficient for recognition in the ELISA assay, but not by the AGE receptor, even after extended incubation with AGE peptides. Both the LDL and the AGE peptides would contain Amadori adducts, providing a mechanism for formation of carboxymethylated LDL, either via glyoxal formation from Amadori adducts on LDL or the AGE peptides, or by direct autoxidation of Amadori adducts on LDL. These autoxidation reactions, and resultant lipid peroxidation, may then lead to the formation of AGEd (carboxymethylated) and peroxidized LDL. Lyons *et al.*[81] recently noted that glycoxidized LDL, i.e. LDL oxidized during glycation under oxidative conditions, was more toxic to cultured retinal capillary endothelial cells and pericytes than either LDL glycated under antioxidative conditions or LDL oxidized under mild conditions, suggesting mechanisms for AGE- or glycoxidation-induced vascular disease in diabetes.

FUTURE DIRECTIONS

The Maillard reaction between carbohydrates and proteins is not a reaction, but a constellation of dendritic and chaotic processes, mediated by a range of carbohydrate, lipid and amino acid reactants. Small differences in metal ion, antioxidant and metabolite concentrations in tissue microenvironments may have profound effects on the chemistry of the reaction. Despite decades of research on the Maillard reaction, the basic structure of the melanoidins in foods are still unknown and the majority of their counterparts in biological systems,

AGEs and glycoxidation products, also remain structurally uncharacterized. Major achievements during the last two decades include: (a) identification of a limited number of useful biomarkers of the progress of the Maillard reaction *in vivo*, and development of chemical and immunochemical methods for their measurement; (b) generation of evidence for the accumulation of Maillard reaction products in tissue proteins with age and for involvement of the Maillard reaction in aging and in the pathogenesis or progression of diseases, including atherosclerosis, diabetes, hemodialysis-associated amyloidosis and Alzheimer's disease; (c) appreciation of the role of nonoxidative and oxidative routes of the reaction and of Maillard reaction products not only as products, but also as initiators and modulators of oxidation chemistry in biological systems; and (d) development of therapeutic approaches for limiting the progress of the Maillard reaction *in vivo*, including studies on the use of dicarbonyl traps and antioxidant supplements.

There is no lack of directions to pursue in future research, only a need to focus on critical goals. These will include: (a) further characterization of reaction products, including studies on crosslink structures, modifications of amino acids other than lysine, and derivatives of lipids in lipoproteins and membranes; (b) identification of characteristic products derived from specific carbohydrate precursors and dicarbonyl intermediates, e.g. ascorbate, de-oxyglucosones and sugar metabolites; (c) understanding the role of oxidative stress in modulation of Maillard reaction damage *in vivo* and the interplay between Maillard reactions of carbohydrates and oxidation of lipids and proteins in aging and in disease; (d) studies on the recognition and degradation of Maillard reaction products in biological systems; and (e) continued studies on the design and evaluation of inhibitors of the Maillard reaction in biological systems for therapeutic intervention in the progress of disease.

During the last two decades, it has become increasingly clear that nonenzymatic Maillard reactions occur ubiquitously in the body, in parallel with enzyme-catalyzed, metabolic reactions. Although the Maillard reaction is scarcely mentioned in major textbooks in biochemistry, the words 'nonenzymatic' and 'Maillard' have now become essential for a modern description of body chemistry. Eventually, with a more complete under-standing of the Maillard reaction, it seems likely that these studies will be integrated into basic and clinical science textbooks and educational materials and that the chemistry of glycation, the Maillard reaction and oxidative stress may well be as important as the intermediary metabolism of carbohydrates and lipids to a comprehensive understanding of human biochemistry.

ACKNOWLEDGMENTS

Research in the author's laboratory was supported by research grants from the National Institute of Diabetes and Digestive and Kidney Disease and from the Juvenile Diabetes Foundation.

REFERENCES

1. J. E. Hodge, *Agric. Food Chem.*, **1**, 928–43 (1953).
2. T. M. Reynolds, *Adv. Food Res.*, **14**, 1–52, 167–283 (1965).
3. P. Thornalley, S. Wolff, J. Crabbe and A. Stern, *Biochim. Biophys. Acta*, **797**, 276–87 (1984).
4. M. Brownlee, *Diabetes*, **43**, 836–41 (1994).
5. H. Vlassara, R. Bucala and L. Striker, *Lab. Invest.*, **70**, 138–51 (1994).
6. B. Halliwell and J. M. C. Gutteridge, *Free Radicals in Biology and Medicine*, 2nd edn, Clarendon Press, Oxford, 1989, 543 pp.
7. S. P. Wolff, Z. Y. Jiang and J. V. Hunt, *Free Rad. Biol. Med.*, **10**, 339–52 (1991).
8. J. W. Baynes, *Diabetes*, **40**, 205–12 (1991).
9. F. Ledl and E. Schleicher, *Angew. Chem.*, **29**, 565–94 (1990).
10. M. S. Feather, *Prog. Food Nutr. Sci.*, **5**, 37–45 (1981).
11. H. Kato, R. K. Cho, A. Okitani and F. Hayase, *Agric. Biol. Chem.*, **51**, 683–9 (1987).
12. B. S. Szwergold, F. Kappler and T. R. Brown, *Science*, **247**, 451–4 (1990).
13. K. J. Wells-Knecht, M. S. Feather and J. W. Baynes, *Arch. Biochem. Biophys.*, **294**, 130–7 (1992).
14. T. Niwa, N. Takeda, H. Yoshizumi, A. Takematsu, M. Ohara, S. Tomiyama and K. Niimura, *Biochem. Biophys. Res. Commun.*, **196**, 837–43 (1993).
15. M. A. Glomb, M. Grissom and V. M. Monnier, in *Maillard Reactions in Chemistry, Food, and Health* (Eds. T. P. Labuza, G. A. Reineccius, V. M. Monnier, J. O'Brien and J. W. Baynes), Royal Society of Chemistry, London, 1994, p. 422A.
16. Y. Konishi, F. Hayase and H. Kato, *Biosci. Biotech. Biochem*, **58**, 1953–55 (1994).
17. T. W. C. Lo, M. E. Westwood, A. C. McLellan, T. Selwood and P. J. Thornalley, *J. Biol. Chem.*, **269**, 32293–8 (1994).
18. B. J. Ortwerth, M. S. Feather and P. R. Olesen, *Exp. Eye Res.*, **47**, 155–68 (1988).
19. J. A. Dunn, M. U. Ahmed, M. H. Murtiashaw, J. M. Richardson, M. D. Walla, S. R. Thorpe and J. W. Baynes, *Biochem*, **29**, 10964–70 (1990).
20. T. Hayashi and M. Namiki, in *Amino-Carbonyl Reactions in Food and Biological Systems* (eds. M. Fujimaki, M. Namiki and H. Kato), Elsevier, Amsterdam, 1986, pp. 29–38.
21. S. P. Wolff and R. T. Dean, *Biochem. J.*, **245**, 243–50 (1987).
22. K. V. Chace, R. Carubelli and R. E. Nordquist, *Arch Biochem. Biophys.*, **288**, 473–80 (1991).
23. M. X. Fu, K. J. Wells-Knecht, S. R. Thorpe and J. W. Baynes, *Diabetes*, **41** (Suppl. 2), 42–8 (1992).
24. M. X. Fu, K. J. Wells-Knecht, J. A. Blackledge, T. J. Lyons, S. R. Thorpe and J. W. Baynes, *Diabetes*, **43**, 676–83 (1994).
25. K. J. Wells-Knecht, D. V. Zyzak, J. E. Litchfield, S. R. Thorpe and J. W. Baynes, *Biochem.*, **34**, 3702–9 (1995).
26. J. A. Blackledge, M. X. Fu, S. R. Thorpe and J. W. Baynes, *J. Org. Chem.*, **58**, 2001–2 (1993).
27. M. E. Westwood, A. C. McLellan and P. J. Thornalley, *J. Biol. Chem.*, **269**, 32299–305 (1994).
28. V. M. Monnier, R. R. Kohn and A. Cerami, *Proc. Natl Acad. Sci. (USA)*, **81**, 583–7 (1984).
29. Y. Nakamura, Y. Horii, T. Nishino, H. Shiiki, Y. Sakaguchi, T. Kagoshima, K. Dohi, Z. Makita, H. Vlassara and R. Bucula, *Am J. Pathol.*, **143**, 1649–56 (1993).

30. N. Araki, N. Ueno, B. Chakrabarti, Y. Morino and S. Horiuchi, *J. Biol. Chem.*, **267**, 10211–12 (1992).
31. Z. Makita, H. Vlassara, A. Cerami and R. Bucala, *J. Biol. Chem.*, **267**, 5133–8 (1992).
32. Z. Makita, H. Vlassara, E. Rayfield, K. Cartwright, E. Friedman, R. Rodby, A. Cerami and R. Bucala, *Science*, **258**, 651–3 (1992).
33. T. Mitsuhashi, H. Nakayama, T. Itoh, S. Kawajima, S. Aoki, T. Atsumi and T. Koike, *Diabetes*, **42**, 826–32 (1993).
34. R. Bucala, Z. Makita, G. Vega, S. Grundy, T. Koschinsky, A. Cerami and H. Vlassara, *Proc. Natl Acad. Sci. (USA)*, **91**, 9441–5 (1994).
35. D. G. Dyer, J. A. Dunn, S. R. Thorpe, K. E. Bailie, T. J. Lyons, D. R. McCance and J. W. Baynes, *J. Clin. Invest.*, **91**, 2463–9 (1993).
36. M. U. Ahmed, J. A. Dunn, M. D. Walla, S. R. Thorpe and J. W. Baynes, *J. Biol. Chem.*, **263**, 8816–21 (1988).
37. F. Hayase, R. H. Nagaraj, S. Miyata, F. G. Njoroge and V. M. Monnier, *J. Biol. Chem.*, **264**, 3758–64 (1989).
38. J. A. Dunn, D. R. McCance, S. R. Thorpe, T. J. Lyons and J. W. Baynes, *Biochem*, **30**, 1205–10 (1991).
39. D. R. Sell and V. M. Monnier, *J. Clin. Invest.*, **85**, 380–4 (1990).
40. P. Odetti, P. Fogarty, D. R. Sell and V. M. Monnier, *Diabetes*, **41**, 153–9 (1992).
41. V. M. Monnier, V. Vishwanath, K. E. Frank, C. A. Elmets, P. Dauchot and R. R. Kohn, *New Engl. J. Med.*, **314**, 403–8 (1986).
42. D. R. Sell and V. M. Monnier, *J. Clin. Invest.*, **85**, 380–4 (1990).
43. D. R. Sell, A. Lapolla, P. Odetti, J. Fogarty and V. M. Monnier, *Diabetes*, **41**, 1286–92 (1992).
44. D. R. McCance, D. G. Dyer, J. A. Dunn, K. E. Bailie, S. R. Thorpe, J. W. Baynes and T. J. Lyons, *J. Clin. Invest.*, **91**, 2470–8 (1993).
45. P. J. Beisswenger, L. L. Moore, T. Brinck-Johnsen and T. J. Curphey, *J. Clin. Invest.*, **92**, 212–17 (1993).
46. K. J. Knecht, J. A. Dunn, K. F. McFarland, D. R. McCance, T. J. Lyons, S. R. Thorpe and J. W. Baynes, *Diabetes*, **40**, 190–6 (1991).
47. K. Nakamura, T. Hasegawa, Y. Fukunaga and K. Ienaga, *J. Chem. Soc., Chem. Commun.*, 992–4 (1992).
48. T. J. Lyons, K. E. Bailie, D. G. Dyer, J. A. Dunn and J. W. Baynes, *J. Clin. Invest.*, **87**, 1910–25 (1991).
49. D. G. Dyer, J. A. Blackledge, B. M. Katz, C. J. Hull, H. D. Adkisson, S. R. Thorpe, T. J. Lyons and J. W. Baynes, *Z. Ernährungswiss*, **30**, 29–45 (1991).
50. R. N. Johnson, P. A. Metcalf and J. R. Baker, *Clin. Chim. Acta*, **127**, 87–95 (1983).
51. J. W. Baynes, N. G. Watkins, C. I. Fisher, C. J. Hull, J. S. Patrick, M. U. Ahmed, J. A. Dunn and S. R. Thorpe, in *The Maillard Reaction in Aging, Diabetes and Nutrition* (eds. J. W. Baynes and V. M. Monnier), Alan R. Liss, New York, 1989, pp. 43–67.
52. J. V. Hunt, M. A. Bottoms and M. J. Mitchinson, *Biochem. J.*, **291**, 529–35 (1993).
53. M. C. Wells-Knecht, S. R. Thorpe and J. W. Baynes. *J. Free Rad. Biol. Med.*, **2**, B16 (1994).
54. J. W. Baynes, *Redox Reports*, **1**, 31–5 (1994).
55. T. Ookawara, N. Kawamura, Y. Kitagawa and N. Taniguchi, *J. Biol. Chem.*, **267**, 18505–10 (1992).
56. S. Grandhee and V. M. Monnier, *J. Biol. Chem.*, **266**, 11649–53 (1991).
57. D. G. Dyer, J. A. Blackledge, S. R. Thorpe and J. W. Baynes, *J. Biol. Chem.*, **266**, 11654–60 (1991).

58. M. X. Fu, S. R. Thorpe and J. W. Baynes, in *Maillard Reactions in Chemistry, Food, and Health* (eds. T. P. Labuza, G. A. Reineccius, V. M. Monnier, J. O'Brien and J. W. Baynes), Royal Society of Chemistry, London, 1994, pp. 95–100.
59. J. W. Baynes, in *Drugs, Diet and Disease*, Vol. 2, *Mechanistic Approaches to Diabetes* (ed. C. Ioannides), Pergamon Press, London (in press).
60. S. Picard, S. Parthasarathy, J. Fruebis and J. L. Witztum, *Proc. Natl Acad. Sci. (USA)*, **89**, 6876–80 (1992).
61. T. J. Lyons, S. R. Thorpe and J. W. Baynes, in *Glucose Metabolism, Diabetes and the Vascular Wall* (eds. N. Ruderman, J. R. Williamson and M. Brownlee), Oxford University Press, New York, 1992, pp. 197–217.
62. T. J. Lyons, *Am. J. Cardiol.*, **71**, 26B-31B (1993).
63. T. J. Lyons, in *Maillard Reactions in Chemistry, Food, and Health*, (eds. T. P. Labuza, G. A. Reineccius, V. M. Monnier, J. O'Brien and J. W. Baynes), Royal Society of Chemistry, London, 1994, pp. 267–73.
64. J. R. Williamson, K. Chang, F. M. Khalid, K. S. Hasan, Y. Ido, T. Kawamura, J. R. Nyengaard, M. Van den Enden, C. Kilo and R. G. Tilton, *Diabetes*, **42**, 801–13 (1993).
65. V. M. Monnier, *J. Gerontol.*, **45**, B105–B111 (1990) — Maillard theory.
66. T. Miyata, O. Oda, R. Inagi, Y. Iida, N. Araki, N. Yamada, S. Horiuchi, N. Taniguchi, K. Maeda and T. Kinoshita, *J. Clin. Invest.*, **93**, 521–8 (1994).
67. M. P. Vitek, K. Bhattacharya, J. M. Glendening, E. Stopa, H. Vlassara, R. Bucala, K. Manogue and A. Cerami, *Proc Natl Acad. Sci. (USA)*, **91**, 4766–70 (1994).
68. S. Horiuchi, N. Araki and Y. Morino, *J. Biol. Chem.*, **266**, 7329–32 (1991).
69. H. Nakayama, S. Taneda, T. Mitsuhashi, S. Kawajima, S. Aoki, Y. Kuroda, K. Misawa, K. Yanagisawa and S. Nakagawa, *J. Immunol. Methods*, **140**, 119–25 (1991).
70. S. Reddy, I. Bichler, K. J. Wells-Knecht, S. R. Thorpe and I. W. Baynes, *Biochem.*, **34**, 10872–8 (1995).
71. K. Takata, S. Horiuchi, N. Araki, M. Shiga, M. Saitoh and Y. Morino, *J. Biol. Chem.*, **263**, 14819–25 (1988).
72. M. S. Brown, S. K. Basu, J. R. Falck, Y. K. Ho and J. L. Goldstein, *J. Supramol. Struct.*, **13**, 67–81 (1980).
73. A. M. Schmidt, R. Mora, R. Cao, S. D. Yan, J. Brett, R. Ramakrishnan, T. C. Tsang, M. Simionescu and D. Stern, *J. Biol. Chem.*, **269**, 9882–8 (1994).
74. J. V. Hunt, C. C. T. Smith and S. P. Wolff, *Diabetes*, **39**, 1420–4 (1990).
75. J. L. Witztum and D. Steinberg, *J. Clin. Invest.*, **88**, 1785–92 (1991).
76. A. Bowie, D. Owens, P. Collins, A. Johnson and G. H. Tomkin, *Atherosclerosis*, **102**, 63–7 (1993).
77. T. J. Lyons, *Diabetic Med.*, **8**, 411–19 (1991).
78. R. Bucala, Z. Makita, T. Koschinsky, A. Cerami and H. Vlassara, *Proc. Natl Acad. Sci. (USA)*, **90**, 6434–8 (1993).
79. H. Vlassara, M. Brownlee and A. Cerami, *Proc. Natl Acad. Sci. (USA)*, **82**, 5588–92 (1985).
80. J. Brett, A. M. Schmidt, S. D. Yan, Y. S. Zou, E. Weidman, D. Pinsky, R. Nowygrod, M. Neeper, C. Przysiecki, A. Shaw, A. Migheli and D. Stern, *Am J. Pathol.*, **143**, 1699–1712 (1993).
81. T. J. Lyons, W. Li, M. C. Wells-Knecht and R. Jokl, *Diabetes*, **43**, 1090–5 (1994).

4

Free Radicals and Glycation Theory

SIMON P. WOLFF

Department of Medicine, University College London Medical School, London

DEFINITION OF TERMS

Glycation, or nonenzymatic glycosylation, is the process by which the aldehyde group of glucose reacts with the amino groups of proteins, DNA or lipids to form Schiff bases and the Amadori adduct. The Maillard reaction is used, here, to define that huge range of reactions that result in the formation of yellow-brown and fluorescent, Maillard, products which occur during or subsequent to glycation. Advanced glycation end-products (AGE) is used interchangeably, as a term, with Maillard products. Since there is no good evidence that the Maillard reaction/AGE formation as defined here is anything but a minor contributory factor to the formation of fluorescence on long-lived proteins *in vivo* I prefer to term those new chemical entities present *in vivo* on long-lived proteins which fluoresce between 400 and 450 nm on excitation around 330–350 nm simply as 'novel fluorophores' (NFPs).

GLUCOSE AUTOXIDATION

Glucose is a reducing sugar because it is capable of enolization to a highly reducing ene-diol from the open-chain, hydroxyaldehyde form of the sugar. The equilibrium reaction leading to ene-diol formation shifts to the right with increasing pH and is the basis of the Fehling solution test for glucose in which the ene-diol reduces cupric to cuprous ion. However, although far slower, this

The Maillard Reaction: Consequences for the Chemical and Life Sciences. Edited by Raphael Ikan
©1996 John Wiley & Sons Ltd

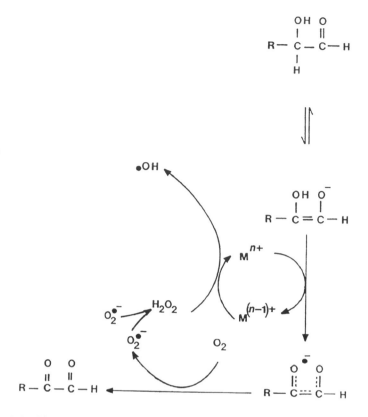

Figure 4.1. Glucose can enolize, reduce transition metal, thereby generating superoxide free radical ($O_2^{\bullet-}$), hydrogen peroxide (H_2O_2) and the hydroxyl radical ($\bullet OH$)

reaction also occurs at physiological pH. *In vitro*, glucose generates hydrogen peroxide (H_2O_2) in a slow process dubbed 'glucose autoxidation' (despite its metal dependency) which also leads to the formation of Girard T-detectable dicarbonyl compounds and hydroxylating agents, probably the hydroxyl radical[1,2]. The postulated chemistry is depicted in Figure 4.1 and the accumulation of H_2O_2 is shown in Figure 4.2. It should be noted that only very low levels of H_2O_2 accumulate (only $5\,\mu M$ H_2O_2 from $100\,mM$ glucose in physiological buffer at $37\,^\circ C$ over an 8-hour period) and that detectable H_2O_2 is the net of formation and consumption of the oxidant. Glucose autoxidation is thus a very sluggish process.

It had been assumed that glucosone was the major detectable dicarbonyl formed by glucose autoxidation. However, the Baynes group has demonstrated that glyoxal is the dominant stable dicarbonyl formed from autoxidizing glucose with arabinose representing the major sugar product.[3] By contrast,

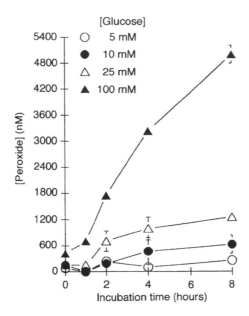

Figure 4.2. Glucose generates H_2O_2 *in vitro*. Glucose was incubated in phosphate buffer at 37°C and the incubation mixture was analyzed for H_2O_2 content using the FOX assay, version 1, as described in Ref. 4

ribulose was the major sugar formed when synthesized glucosone was incubated in buffer. The observation that glyoxal and arabinose are the major products detectable in solutions of autoxidizing glucose implies either that glucose autoxidation proceeds via a mechanism different to that outlined above (the ene-diol might migrate through the molecule prior to its oxidation, for example) or that hydroxyl radical attack on glucose molecules leads to chain reactions that result in glyoxal formation. The latter explanation is not unreasonable since it is known that the reaction of ferrous ions and H_2O_2 with polyol sugars gives rise to extensive chain reactions involving carbohydrate free radicals[4]. I speculate that H_2O_2 initially formed together with small amounts of glucosone further reacts with transition metal initiating free radical chain reactions which lead to glyoxal and arabinose as dominant, but secondary, products. This type of reaction is likely, however, to occur only in pure solutions of glucose. In more complex environments, such as *in vivo*, or even when glucose is incubated in the presence of protein, then secondary oxidants formed from H_2O_2 would react with other molecules, such as amino acid side chains, rather than bulk solution glucose. Glyoxal would be formed in far smaller yields under these circumstances. Resolution of these questions requires careful experimentation and, ultimately, identification of glyoxal *in vivo*.

THE PARADOXICAL ROLE OF TRANSITION METALS IN GLUCOSE AUTOXIDATION

Whatever the precise mechanism, there is no doubt that glucose is a low-grade oxidizing agent which gives rise to H_2O_2, hydroxylating agents and reactive dicarbonyl compounds. The process of glucose autoxidation can only be inhibited by the inclusion of agents that chelate transition metals tightly and thus prevent oxidation of the ene-diol. However, the role of transition metal in this *in vitro* process is somewhat paradoxical. The rate of glucose autoxidation is limited by the availability of transition metal and rate of enolization. Most physiological buffers contain trace levels of iron and copper (less than $1 \mu M$) which tend to be higher than the concentration of ene-diol. For example, a 25 mM solution of glucose may contain only 25 nM ene-diol versus 500 nM total transition metal. This means, in effect, that the system is already saturated with respect to transition metal and that the ene-diol will oxidize as fast as it is formed. Removal of the metal by chelation dramatically shows ene-diol oxidation whereas addition of further metal has no stimulatory effect upon ene-diol oxidation. However, the addition of further metal will lessen accumulation of H_2O_2 in the reaction mixture, as this undergoes accelerated degradation by metal to form hydroxylating agents. Under these circumstances, measurement of H_2O_2 may lead to the erroneous conclusion that metals inhibit glucose autoxidation. The net effect of adding further metal would be, however, to increase the production of secondary oxidation products from glucose.

The role of glucose autoxidation *in vivo* is unknown but its contribution to *in vitro* processes is undisputed. For example, the well-known conformational alterations that occur when bovine serum albumin (BSA) is exposed to glucose under physiological conditions *in vitro* are inhibited by the metal chelating agents diethylenetriaminepentaacetic acid (DETAPAC) or ethylenediaminetetraacetic acid and hydroxyl radical scavengers[5]. Hydroxyl radicals or similar oxidizing species cause the protein to become fragmented (Figure 4.3). Oxidative reactions are thus critical for the production of glucose-induced protein alterations.[6] The rate of glucose autoxidation is slow, but the amounts of dicarbonyls and oxidizing agents formed over the typical time courses of *in vitro* studies of glucose and proteins (days to weeks) are in the range consistent with protein damage and modification by this process. Incubation of glucose with any biological material is far more complicated than the simple addition of glucose to free amino groups. Indeed, transition metal catalyzed processes accompanying the incubation of proteins with glucose also contribute to the formation of Maillard products. If protein is incubated with glucose in the presence of DETAPAC the browning and crosslinking process is inhibited.[7] It should be noted, furthermore, that attempting to render glucose/protein incubation mixtures anaerobic is unlikely to block glucose autoxidation. Air-

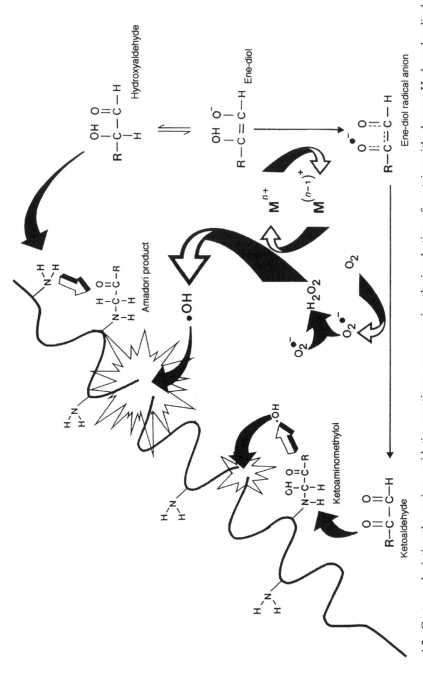

Figure 4.3. Cartoon depicting the various oxidative reactions accompanying the incubation of proteins with glucose. Hydroxyl radical cleavage of protein is depicted as well as the reaction of dicarbonyls (ketoaldehyde) with protein amino groups. It is postulated that such adducts also undergo metal-catalyzed reactions, causing localized protein damage

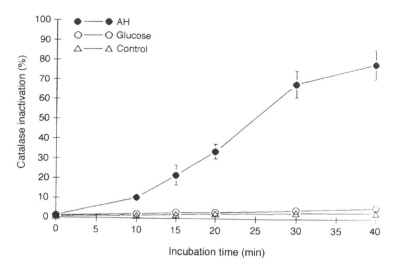

Figure 4.4. A comparison of H_2O_2 fluxes induced within the erythrocyte by ascorbate (AH) and glucose. Erythrocytes were incubated with glucose and ascorbate in the presence of aminotriazole, which inactivates catalase only in the presence of a flux of H_2O_2. Residual catalase activity in the cells was then taken as an index of the H_2O_2 flux

saturated buffers contain approximately 200 μM oxygen and it is not feasible to reduce this level to less than 1 μM which would be the minimum required for glucose autoxidation to be noticeably inhibited.

DOES GLUCOSE AUTOXIDATION OCCUR *IN VIVO*?

Doubts about the importance of glucose autoxidation *in vivo* come from several considerations. It is not clear whether there is any 'decompartmentalized', catalytically active transition metal *in vivo*. If there is such a pool of metal available it is highly unlikely that glucose autoxidation would contribute greatly to any oxidative stress. Decompartmentalized transition metal would, of course, contribute to a general oxidative stress since it would cause the oxidation of other molecules, such as vitamin C, thiols and lipids, which would be likely to occur far more rapidly than glucose autoxidation. For example, when the erythrocyte is exposed to physiological levels of ascorbic acid, an ene-diol, *in vitro*, there is a flux of H_2O_2 through the cell which is mediated by catalytically active, chelatable transition metal, probably copper.[8] This flux of H_2O_2, induced by physiological levels of ascorbate, is more than 100 times as fast as that produced when the erythrocyte is exposed to a level of glucose representative of hyperglycaemia (Figure 4.4). Furthermore, glucosone, if it is formed *in vivo*, is likely to be present in extremely small amounts and react with protein amino groups to form adducts probably indistinguishable from the Amadori product.

GLUCOSE ONLY WEAKLY STIMULATES CO-OXIDATIONS *IN VITRO*

When molecules are incubated with glucose *in vitro* a variety of transition metal-catalyzed processes can be expected to occur. For example, low-density lipoprotein (LDL) has been shown to be massively peroxidized when exposed to glucose *in vitro*[9–11] but the rate of oxidation of LDL *in vitro* under basal conditions is only slightly accelerated by glucose. Transition metal present in buffer will catalyze the oxidation of lipid more rapidly than of glucose so that the contribution of glucose autoxidation to lipid oxidation is generally minor. Conditions have to be severely manipulated so that any such increased oxidation stimulated by glucose can be shown. Similar considerations apply when thiol-rich proteins, such as the lens crystallins, are incubated with glucose *in vitro*.[12] Glucose will stimulate crystallin crosslinking and thiol oxidation, and this process is inhibitable by metal chelators. However, crystallin oxidation by transition metal is already very rapid[13] and glucose makes only a very minor contribution to protein oxidation. If there is decompartmentalized metal available for glucose autoxidation *in vivo* then it is obvious that other oxidative processes will occur at rates orders of magnitude faster than glucose autoxidation. Furthermore, it is likely that glucose would enter into this oxidative stress through other routes.

AMADORI ADDUCT OXIDATION

Work by Baynes and colleagues has shown that the Amadori adduct itself is also able to oxidize, similarly catalyzed by transition metals, leading to the release of erythronic acid and the formation of carboxymethylated lysine residues (Figure 4.5).[14,15] Baynes and colleagues have studied skin collagen CML formation in relation to the complications of diabetes and found that CML levels are twice as high in skin collagen from diabetics compared with age-matched nondiabetics[16] and that the level of skin CML correlates positively with the presence of retinopathy and nephropathy, correcting for age.[17] CML, although present only in trace concentrations (less than 1% of total lysine groups), is strongly indicative of the hypothesis that transition metal-catalyzed oxidations occur *in vivo*. Thus CML accumulation may indicate either an accumulation of oxidizable substrate (i.e. the Amadori adduct in diabetes and ageing) and/or an increased level of transition metal in a form capable of catalyzing oxidation. However, this process is likely to be slow

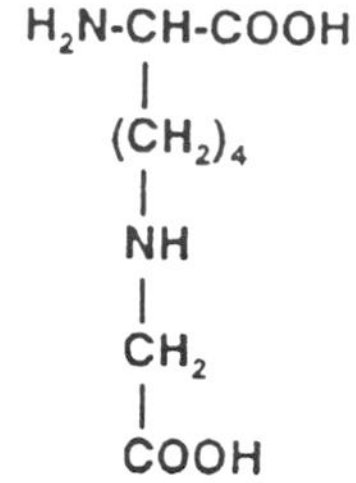

$$\begin{array}{c} \text{H}_2\text{N-CH-COOH} \\ | \\ (\text{CH}_2)_4 \\ | \\ \text{NH} \\ | \\ \text{CH}_2 \\ | \\ \text{COOH} \end{array}$$

N^{ε}-(Carboxymethyl)lysine

Figure 4.5. The structure of carboxymethyllysine

compared to the very fast oxidation of other reducing agents. Baynes refers to CML as a biomarker for oxidative processes. In my view, the identification of CML *in vivo* is perhaps the first evidence, albeit indirect, that transition metals must be available in a form *in vivo* that can catalyze adventitious oxidation. For reasons given below, however, the precise route by which CML forms *in vivo* remains unclear.

Baynes and colleagues[18] have shown, for example, that CML is also able to form from ascorbic acid, raising the possibility that the Amadori adduct may not be the sole source of CML formation *in vivo*. Kawakishi and colleagues have contributed to uncertainty concerning the oxidative fate of the Amadori adduct by showing that glucosone is a further major product of *in vitro* Amadori adduct oxidation.[19] Glucosone accumulation appears to be greater at higher pH values, such as in the 'fructosamine' assay,[20] suggesting reversibility of the Amadori adduct to yield open-chain, oxidizable carboydrate. The group of Monnier has also shown that CML is an important product of the *in vitro* reaction of glyoxal with lysine, supporting the possibility that CML may be a glucose autoxidation product with proteins and not form via the mechanism, originating from fructoselyine, the Amadori product, originally proposed by Baynes.[21]

PENTOSIDINE

Further work by the groups of Baynes and Monnier has led to the identification of an important NFP on collagen termed 'pentosidine'. Pentosidine is a highly fluorescent crosslinking compound derived from a pentose, arginine and

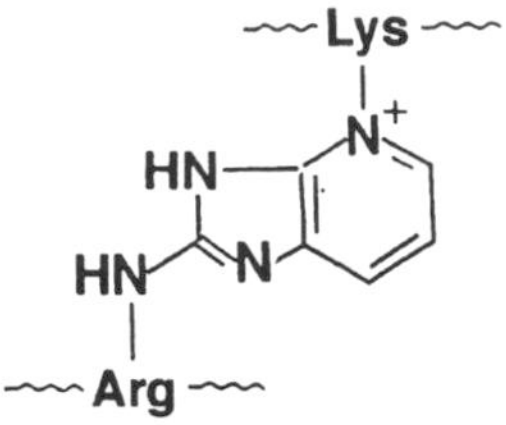

Figure 4.6. The structure of pentosidine

lysine[22,23] in an imidazo(4,5,6)pyridinium ring (Figure 4.6). It can be formed from glucose, fructose and even ascorbate by a sequence of transition metal-catalyzed oxidation and decarboxylation reactions.[24,25] Pentosidine increases with age and more so in diabetes but is present only in extremely small amounts; less than 1 in 200 000 lens crystallin lysine residues is part of a pentosidine molecule. This suggests that pentosidine itself is unlikely to play any pathological role in the later complications of long-term diabetes mellitus. Nevertheless, skin collagen pentosidine correlates positively with the presence of retinopathy and nephropathy in the diabetic patient and accounts for as much as 40% of total NFP in the lens.[26]

ROUTES TO PENTOSIDINE FORMATION

Although it is natural to believe that fluorescent molecules in diabetes would be derived from glucose reactions with protein as a result of hyperglycaemia, evidence suggests that in the case of human cataract the major route to fluorophore and pentosidine formation is the reaction of ascorbic acid with crystallins.[27] Increased oxidation of ascorbate to dehydroascorbate and 2,3-diketogulonate followed by decarboxylation to xylosone is ostensibly the route of formation of pentosidine in human cataract. The formation of pentosidine under these circumstances would thus appear to be the result of a catastrophic failure of biological defence systems. The rate of ascorbate oxidation must be increased and/or the rate of reduction of dehydroascorbate by glutathione and ascorbate reductase to the reduced form must be decreased. There must also be a failure of the glyoxalase system to trap the ketoaldehydes 2,3-diketogulonate and xylosone. If ascorbate oxidation does contribute to pentosidine formation *in vivo* then it can be freely speculated that there must be vast ascorbate oxidation accompanying the formation of small amounts of pentosidine. This again raises the possibility that NFP, such as pentosidine, or protein-bound oxidation products, such as CML, are indirect measures of the rate of transition metal- and oxygen-dependent oxidations *in vivo*. Ascorbate oxidation is known to be increased in human diabetes.[28] Careful study of pentosidine levels in disease has shown that pentosidine levels of plasma proteins are elevated not

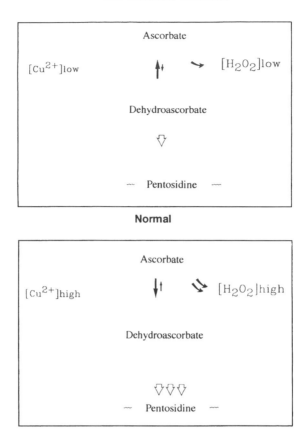

Figure 4.7. Elevated pentosidine formation from ascorbate and decompartmentalized copper ion in diabetes mellitus

merely in diabetes (2.5-fold elevation) but are greatly increased also in uraemia associated with end-stage renal disease (23-fold elevation).[29] Given that blood sugar levels are not elevated in uraemia it follows that factors other than hyperglycaemia and glucose-derived modifications are responsible for pentosidine elevation in uraemia, and, by extension, perhaps also in diabetes. Monnier has hypothesized that the increased level of dehydroascorbate in diabetes mellitus[30] could provide an explanation for the increased levels of pentosidine in diabetes mellitus as well as in uraemia. Figure 4.7 shows the speculative relationships that may occur between decompartmentalized copper, ascorbate and pentosidine *in vivo* in the presence and absence of diabetes. It is proposed that there is elevated decompartmentalized copper ion which increases the rate of ascorbate oxidation and consequently pentosidine.

COPPER AND THE ALDOSE REDUCTASE INHIBITORS

Further indirect evidence for such transition metal-catalyzed oxidation in diabetes mellitus has come from an animal model of diabetes. Rodents fed a diet containing high levels of galactose develop cataract which is morphologically and biochemically similar to cataract found in diabetes and which can also be blocked by a group of drugs collectively termed the 'aldose reductase inhibitors'. The aldose reductase inhibitor Sorbinil blocks lens protein NFP development in galactosaemia[31] and lessens the accumulation of pentosidine.[32] A possible explanation for this effect of sorbinil is offered by our finding that some of these compounds bind free copper ions and can thereby block copper-catalyzed ascorbate oxidation.[33] Several of the aldose reductase inhibitors prevent H_2O_2 formation in erythrocytes exposed to physiological ascorbate (Ou and Wolff, unpublished). Aldose reductase inhibitors reverse the depletion of plasma ascorbic acid found in experimental diabetes which would be consistent with a transition metal-binding effect of the drugs and further suggest abnormalities in copper compartmentalization in diabetes.[34] It seems unavoidable, to this author at least, that transition metals occupy a shadowy background in all studies related to the physiology of Maillard reactions.

This speculation is partially supported by the observation that many physiologically abundant oxidizable molecules such as vitamin C and unsaturated fatty acids are efficient producers of NFPs and crosslinking agents *in vitro*, when their oxidation is permitted by the presence of oxygen and trace amounts of transition metals.[35–38] For example, NFP development in collagen, lens crystallin and albumin is much more extensive with ascorbate and arachidonic acid than with glucose, and in these cases is similarly inhibited by metal-chelating agents.[39] *In vitro*, at least, browning reactions caused by a variety of aldehyde-forming molecules are dependent upon the presence of trace amounts of transition metals which catalyze the oxidative reactions required.

CAN AGEs LEAD TO OXIDATION WITHOUT METALS?

The collective evidence would seem to suggest that oxidative reactions accompanying hyperglycaemia, glycation and the Maillard reaction imply elevated decompartmentalized transition metal *in vivo*. Maillard and other oxidation products possibly derived from glucose *in vivo* would then serve as no more than biomarkers of parallel oxidative processes involving thiols, ascorbate and lipids. There have been various ambitious attempts, however, to suggest that oxidative stress *in vivo* is consequent upon glycation and the Maillard reaction. For example, Cerami and coworkers have recently compared the ability of phosphatidylethanolamine (PE: one free amino group) and phosphatidylcholine (PC: no amino groups) to generate NFP and lipid oxidation products in the presence of glucose and EDTA.[40] Their conclusion that lipid oxidation progressed more rapidly in the PE preparation than in the PC preparation because the free amino group formed an 'AGE' would be more convincing if it could be shown that (a) EDTA blocked transition metal-catalyzed lipid peroxidation, rather than just slowing it down, and (b) PE does not contain a higher proportion of very peroxidizable polyunsaturated fatty acid (PUFA) than PC. Experiments in our lab suggest, in fact, that EDTA, like DETAPAC, only inhibit metal-catalyzed reactions. Further, our purchased batches of PE inevitably contain more PUFA than commercial PC, rendering them more susceptible to peroxidation by any initiating agent.

AGE, OXIDATIVE STRESS AND ARTEFACTS

It is critical to have well-defined reaction systems before trying to reach conclusions about reaction chemistry. In this context, it seems premature to attempt to assess the potential role of AGE and proposed AGE receptors in cellular oxidative processes.[41,42] This is, of course, an expanding and important field but appears very poorly characterized. For example, one of the early crosslinking and fluorescent AGEs found in hydrolysates of *in vitro* glycated protein was identified as 2-furoyl-4[5]-[2-furanyl]-1-*H*-imidazole (FFI).[43] This compound was suggested to be relevant to protein crosslinking and fluorescence *in vivo* since a specific macrophage receptor (distinct from the well-known 'scavenger' receptor) had been identified which appeared to recognize proteins which had been exposed to glucose *in vitro* or to which FFI was attached.[44] However, FFI is not formed as a result of rearrangements of the Amadori adduct, as originally speculated, but is produced as an *in vitro* artefact by the condensation of furosine (produced when glycated protein is hydrolysed to amino acids) with the ammonia used to neutralize the hydrolysates.[45] FFI is not present *in vivo*[46,47] and a great deal of work on this molecule (in particular, evidence relating to specific receptors for the molecule and the selectivity of antibodies raised to test its *in vivo* presence) needs to be reappraised. The specificity of antibodies raised against proteins incubated with glucose *in vitro* is not known so that use of the antibody to identify AGE proteins in tissue preparations is not compelling.[48]

SUMMARY AND CONCLUSIONS

This selective review of the current state of free radical glycation theory ends with a conclusion that much more needs to be known about the role of transition metals in this chemistry. Glucose autoxidation yielding dicarbonyl compounds such as glyoxal and, probably, glucosone, pentosidine and CML is a complex metal-catalyzed process that occurs *in vitro* and is important when molecules are incubated with glucose *in vitro*. Co-oxidation of the molecules probably contributes heavily to molecular alterations associated with glycation. The process thus cannot be ignored although it can be minimized by the metal-chelating agents. *In vitro*, formation of the Amadori adduct is also associated with the formation of CML and glucosone.

In vivo, glucose autoxidation may also proceed if transition metal is available, but the rate of this process will be infinitely slow compared to the metal-catalyzed oxidation of thiols, ascorbate, lipids and other easily oxidized materials. Glucose autoxidation is thus unlikely to contribute to oxidative stress although it may provide small fluxes of dicarbonyls. Pentosidine and CML are also formed *in vivo*, but it is entirely unclear how these compounds are formed. Pentosidine may well be derived via ascorbic acid oxidation (a conclusion based largely upon the elevation of pentosidine in uraemia), whereas CML may be formed either from the Amadori adduct or ascorbate oxidation. The presence of CML and pentosidine strongly suggests a role for metal-catalyzed oxidative processes *in vivo*. The correlation of these materials with the presence of diabetic tissue damage can be taken to indicate a role for oxidative stress in the diabetic complications. Future research should focus on identification of *in vivo* pathways to these biomarkers.

REFERENCES

1. S. P. Wolff and R. T. Dean, Glucose autoxidation and protein oxidation: the role of autoxidative glycosylation in diabetes mellitus and ageing, *Biochem. J.*, **245**, 243–50 (1987).
2. Z.-Y. Jiang, A. C. S. Woollard and S. P. Wolff, Hydrogen peroxide production during experimental protein glycation, *FEBS Lett.*, **268**, 69–71 (1990).
3. K. J. Wells-Knecht, D. V. Zyzak, J. F. Litchfield, S. R. Thorpe and J. W. Baynes, Mechanism of autoxidative glycosylation — identification of glyoxal and arabinose as intermediates in the autoxidative modification of proteins by glucose, *Biochem*, **34**, 3702–9 (1995).
4. S. P. Wolff, Ferrous ion oxidation in the presence of the ferric ion indicator xylenol orange for the measurement of hydroperoxides: the 'FOX' assay, in *Methods in Enzymology. Oxygen Radicals in Biological Systems*, Part C, Vol. 233, Academic Press, New York, 1994, pp. 182–9.
5. J. V. Hunt, R. T. Dean and S. P. Wolff, Hydroxyl radical production and autoxidative glycosylation: glucose autoxidation as the cause of protein damage in the experimental glycation model of diabetes mellitus and ageing, *Biochem. J.*, **256**, 205–12 (1988).
6. S. P. Wolff and R. T. Dean, Aldehydes and ketoaldehydes in the non-enzymatic glycosylation of proteins, *Biochem. J.*, **249**, 617–19 (1988).
7. M. X. Fu, K. J. Wells-Knecht, J. A. Blackledge, T. J. Lyons, S. R. Thorpe and J. W. Baynes, Glycation, glycoxidation, and cross-linking of collagen by glucose-kinetics, mechanisms, and inhibition of late stages of the Maillard reaction, *Diabetes*, **43**, 676–83 (1994).

8. P. Ou and S. P. Wolff, Erythrocyte catalase inactivation (H_2O_2 production) by ascorbic acid and glucose in the presence of aminotriazole: role of transition metals, relevance to diabetes, *Biochem. J.*, **303**, 935–40 (1994).

9. J. V. Hunt, C. C. T. Smith and S. P. Wolff, Autoxidative glycosylation and possible involvement of peroxides and free radicals in LDL modification by glucose, *Diabetes*, **39**, 1420–4 (1990).

10. T. Sakurai, S. Kimura, M. Nakano and H. Kimura, Oxidative modification of glycated low density lipoprotein in the presence of iron, *Biochem. Biophys. Res. Commun.*, **177**, 433–9 (1991).

11. M. Kawamura, J. W. Heinecke and A. Chait, Pathophysiological concentrations of glucose promote oxidative modification of low-density-lipoprotein by a superoxide-dependent pathway, *J. Clin. Invest.*, **94**, 771–8 (1994).

12. B. Li and R. Carubelli, The role of glycation and autoxidation on crystallin aggregation, *Redox Report*, **1**, 205–12 (1995).

13. S. P. Wolff and J. V. Hunt, Hydrogen peroxide production by crystallin: evidence for a site-specific mechanism of oxidative damage in cataract, *Free Radical Biol. Med.*, **13**, 319–23 (1992).

14. M. U. Ahmed, S. R. Thorpe and J. W. Baynes, Identification of N-carboxymethyllysine as a degradation product of fructoselysine in glycated protein, *J. Biol. Chem.*, **261**, 4889–94 (1986).

15. J. W. Baynes, Role of oxidative stress in development of complications in diabetes, *Diabetes*, **40**, 205–12 (1991).

16. D. G. Dyer, J. A. Dunn, S. R. Thorpe, K. E. Bailie, T. J. Lyons, D. R. McCance and J. W. Baynes, Accumulation of Maillard reaction products in skin collagen in diabetes and aging, *J. Clin. Invest.*, **91**, 2463–9 (1993).

17. D. R. McCance, D. G. Dyer, J. A. Dunn, K. E. Bailie, S. R. Thorpe, J. W. Baynes and T. J. Lyons, Maillard reaction products and their relation to complications in insulin dependent diabetes mellitus, *J. Clin. Invest.*, **91**, 2470–6 (1993).

18. J. A. Dunn, M. U. Ahmed, M. H. Murtiashaw, J. M. Richardson, M. D. Walla, S. R. Thorpe and J. W. Baynes, Reaction of ascorbate with lysine and protein under autoxidising conditions: formation of N-(carboxymethyl)lysine by reaction between lysine and products of autoxidation of ascorbate, *Biochem.*, **29**, 10964–70 (1990).

19. R. Z. Cheng, K. Uchida and S. Kawakishi, Selective oxidation of histidine residues in proteins or peptides through the copper (II)-catalyzed autoxidation of glucosone, *Biochem. J.*, **285**, 667–71 (1992).

20. J. R. Baker, D. V. Zyzak, S. R. Thorpe and J. W. Baynes, Chemistry of the fructosamine assay — D-glucosone is the product of oxidation of Amadori compounds, *Clin. Chem.*, **40**, 1950–5 (1994).

21. M. A. Glomb and V. M. Monnier, Mechanism of protein modification by glyoxal and glycolaldehyde, *J. Biol. Chem.*, **270**, 10017–26 (1995).

22. D. R. Sell and V. M. Monnier, Structure elucidation of a senescence crosslink from human extracellular matrix: implication of pentoses in the aging process, *J. Biol. Chem.*, **264**, 21597–602 (1989).

23. D. R. Sell and V. M. Monnier, End-stage renal disease and diabetes catalyze the formation of a pentose-derived cross link from aging human collagen, *J. Biol. Chem.*, **85**, 380–84 (1990).

24. S. K. Grandhee and V. M. Monnier, Mechanism of formation of the Maillard protein crosslink pentosidine: glucose, fructose and ascorbate as pentosidine precursors, *J. Biol. Chem.*, **266**, 11649–53 (1991).

25. D. G. Dyer, J. A. Blackledge, S. R. Thorpe and J. W. Baynes, Formation of pentosidine during non-enzymatic browning of proteins by glucose: identification of glucose and other carbohydrates as possible precursors of pentosidine *in vivo*. *J. Biol. Chem.*, **266**, 11654–60 (1991).

26. D. R. Sell, A. Lapolla, P. Odetti, J. Fogarty and V. M. Monnier, Pentosidine formation in skin correlates with severity of complications in individuals with long-standing insulin-dependent diabetes mellitus, *Diabetes*, **41**, 1286–92 (1992).

27. R. H. Nagaraj, D. R. Dell, M. Prabhakaram, B. J. Ortwerth and V. M. Monnier, High correlation between pentosidine protein crosslinks and pigmentation implicates ascorbate oxidation in human lens sensescence and cataractogenesis, *Proc. Natl Acad. Sci.*, **88**, 10257–61 (1991).

28. A. Sinclair, A. J. Girling, L. Gray, L. Leguen, C. Lunec and A. H. Barnett, Disturbed handling of ascorbic acid in diabetic patients with and without microangiopathy during high dose ascorbate supplementation, *Diabetologia*, **34**, 171–5 (1991).

29. P. Odetti, J. Fogarty, D. R. Sell and V. M. Monnier, Chromatographic quantitation of plasma and erythrocyte pentosidine in diabetic and uremic subjects, *Diabetes*, **41**, 153–9 (1992).

30. I. B. Chatterjee and A. Banerjee, Estimation of dehydroascorbic acid in blood of diabetic patients, *Anal. Biochem.*, **98**, 368–74 (1979).

31. R. Nagaraj and V. M. Monnier, Non-tryptophan fluorescence and high molecular weight protein formation in lens crystallins of rats with chronic galactosaemia: prevention by the aldose reductase inhibitor sorbinil, *Exp. Eye Res.*, **51**, 411–18 (1990).

32. R. H. Nagaraj, M. Prabhakaram, B. J. Ortwerth and V. M. Monnier, Suppression of pentosidine formation in galactosaemic rat lens by an inhibitor of aldose reductase, *Diabetes*, **43**, 580–6.

33. Z.-Y. Jiang, L.-Z. Qiong, J. W. Eaton, J. V. Hunt, W. H. Koppenol and S. P. Wolff, Spirohydantoin inhibitors of aldose reductase inhibit iron- and copper-catalysed ascorbate oxidation *in vitro*, *Biochem. Pharmacol.*, **42**, 1273–8 (1991).

34. K. Yue, S. McLennan, E. Fisher, S. Heffernan, C. Capogreco, G. R. Ross and J. R. Turtle, Ascorbic acid metabolism and polyol pathway in diabetes, *Diabetes*, **38**, 257–61 (1989).

35. J. M. C. Gutteridge, Age pigments and free radicals: fluorescent lipid complexes formed by iron- and copper-containing proteins, *Biochim. Biophys. Acta*, **834**, 144–8 (1985).

36. B. J. Ortwerth, M. S. Feather and P. R. Olesen, The precipitation and crosslinking of lens crystallins by ascorbic acid, *Exp. Eye Res.*, **47**, 155–68 (1988).

37. E. Koller, O. Quehenberger, G. Jurgens, O. S. Wolfbeis and H. Esterbauer, Investigation of human plasma low density lipoprotein by three-dimensional fluorescence spectroscopy, *FEBS Lett.*, **198**, 229–34 (1986).

38. B. J. Ortwerth and P. R. Olesen, Ascorbic acid-induced crosslinking of lens proteins: evidence supporting a Maillard reaction, *Biochim. Biophys. Acta*, **956**, 10–22 (1988).

39. S. P. Wolff and J. V. Hunt, Is glucose the sole source of tissue browning in diabetes mellitus?, *FEBS Lett.*, **269**, 258–60 (1990).

40. R. Bucala, Z. Makita, T. Koschinsky, A. Cerami and H. Vlassara, Lipid advanced glycosylation: pathway for lipid oxidation *in vivo*, *Proc. Natl Acad. Sci. (USA)*, **90**, 6434–8 (1993).

41. R. Bucala, H. Vlassara and A. Cerami, Advanced glycosylation endproducts — role in diabetic and non-diabetic vascular disease, *Drug Dev. Res.*, **32**, 77–89 (1994).

42. J. L. Wautier, M. P. Wautier, A. M. Schmidt, G.M. Anderson, O. Hori, C. Zoukorian, L. Capron, O. Chappey, S. D. Yan, J. Brett, P. J. Guillausseau and D. Stern, Advanced glycation end-products (AGEs) on the surface of diabetic erythrocytes bind to the vessel wall via a specific receptor inducing oxidant stress in the vasculature — a link between surface associated AGEs and diabetic complications, *Proc. Natl Acad. Sci.*, **91**, 7742–6 (1994).

43. S. Pongor, P. C. Ulrich, F. A. Bencsath and A. Cerami, Aging of proteins: isolation and identification of a fluorescent chromophore from the reaction of polypeptides with glucose, *Proc. Natl Acad. Sci. (USA)*, **81**, 2684–8 (1984).

44. H. Vlassara, M. Brownlee and A. Cerami, Novel macrophage receptor for glucose-modified proteins is distinct from previously described scavenger receptors, *J. Exp. Med.*, **164**, 1301–9 (1986).

45. F. G. Njoroge, A. A. Fernandes and V. M. Monnier, Mechanism of formation of the putative advanced glycosylation end product and protein crosslink 2-(2-furoyl)-4(5)-(2-furanyl)-*H*-imidazole, *J. Biol. Chem.*, **263**, 10646–52 (1988).

46. S. Horiuchi, M. Shiga, N. Araki, K. Takata, M. Saitoh and Y. Morino, Evidence against *in vivo* presence of 2-(2-furoyl)-4(5)-(2-furanyl)-1*H*-imidazole, a major fluorescent advanced end product generated by non-enzymatic glycosylation, *J. Biol. Chem.*, **263**, 18821–6 (1990).

47. A. Lapolla, C. Gerhardinger, B. Pelli, A. Sturaro, E. Del Favero, P. Traldi, G. Crepaldi and D. Fedele, Absence of brown product FFI in nondiabetic and diabetic rat collagen, *Diabetes*, **39**, 57–61 (1990).

48. Z. Makita, H. Vlassara, A. Cerami and R. Bucala, Immunochemical detection of advanced glycosylation endproducts *in vivo*, *J. Biol. Chem.*, **267**, 5133–8 (1992).

5

Scavenging of Active Oxygen by Melanoidins

FUMITAKA HAYASE

Department of Agricultural Chemistry, Meiji University, Kawasaki, Japan

The amino-carbonyl reaction is one of the most important reactions in chemical changes of food components during storage and processing of foods. This reaction is known to proceed nonenzymatically, progressing also *in vivo* as well as in soil. The nonenzymatic browning reaction, or the Maillard reaction, has been understood as a universal reaction occurring in nature. Melanoidins, which are the final products of the reaction, are nitrogen-containing polymeric substances that decompose with difficulty. Man consumes melanoidins daily in browning foods. In this article, the formation, chemical structure, physiological effects and scavenging of active oxygen species of melanoidins are discussed.

FORMATION OF MELANOIDINS

The formation mechanism of melanoidins is complex because many reactants, such as osones, unsaturated osones, furfurals, pyrrolyl aldehydes (pyrraline), carbonyl compounds generated by cleavage of reducing sugars, and various amino compounds are involved (Namiki, 1988; Hayashi and Namiki, 1986a, 1986b; Hayase and Kato, 1986, 1994). The formation of melanoidins is estimated to be affected by various factors such as types of reducing sugars and amino compounds, their concentrations, types of catalysts and buffers, reaction temperatures and time, pH, reactivity in water and presence of oxygen and metals.

Under neutral to alkaline pH, melanoidins have been reported to be formed via pyrazinium radicals by cleavage of compounds composed of two or three

The Maillard Reaction: Consequences for the Chemical and Life Sciences. Edited by Raphael Ikan
©1995 John Wiley & Sons Ltd

carbons by splitting of reducing sugars (Hayashi and Namiki, 1986a, 1986b). Under neutral to acidic pH, osones and furfurals are considered to be involved in the formation of melanoidins, which were observed from the formation of cleaved products under alkaline conditions. Also observed were heterocyclic compounds containing six carbons derived from glucose under acidic conditions. The products were obtained under neutral pH, using glucose–butylamine reaction systems (Hayase and Kato, 1985, 1994).

Melanoidins dealt with in this article comprise the nondialyzable ones, which are formed by heating at approximately 100 °C in weak acidic conditions, unless otherwise stated. Melanoidins are high molecular weight compounds showing normal absorption and having no maximum absorption in the UV–visible region. Lignins, tannins, melanins, caramel and humins are organic compounds known to be similar in chemical properties to melanoidins. These compounds, which are generally classified as poikilopolymers, are difficult to identify because of the polydisperse system effect on molecular weight and electric properties (Piattell, 1961; Gomyo and Miura, 1983). Since humins in poikilopolymers are similar to melanoidins in chemical structure, the Maillard reaction probably plays an important role in the formation of humins (Benzing-Purdie *et al.*, 1986; Ikan *et al.*, 1990).

Evidence that molecules of melanoidins are distributed as a polydisperse system has been studied to some extent. Homma *et al.* (1982) detected 14 bands of melanoidins obtained from the reaction system of glucose and glycine (abbreviated as Glc–Gly MEL in this section) by isoelectric electrophoresis at pH 2.7–3.3. O'Reilly (1983) has reported 20 bands at pH 2.5–4.0 and 16 bands at pH 4.0–6.0 in Maillard reaction products formed from xylose and glycine.

CHEMICAL STRUCTURE OF MELANOIDINS

Benzing-Purdie *et al.* (Benzing-Purdie and Ratcliffe, 1986; Benzing-Purdie *et al.*, 1983) have tried to analyze Xyl–Gly (^{15}N) MEL by ^{15}N-CP-MAS NMR. They suggested that signals in the regions of 60–150 ppm are due to secondary amide, pyrrole and indole-like nitrogens.

The authors also analyzed Glc–Gly MEL enriched with ^{13}C or ^{15}N before and after ozonolysis, by ^{13}C- and ^{15}N-CP-MAS NMR (Hayase *et al.*, 1986). Figure 5.1 shows that the signals of Glc–Gly MEL by ^{13}C-CP-MAS NMR could be grouped into six major regions: saturated carbons joined to carbon or nitrogen atoms, or methyl carbons (10–50 ppm, peak I), saturated carbons bound with oxygen or nitrogen (60–75 ppm, peak II), unsaturated or aromatic carbons (105–115 ppm, peak III and 130–140 ppm, peak IV), and amide or carboxyl carbons (170–180 ppm, peak V) and carbonyl carbons (190–205 ppm, peak VI). Peaks I, II and V were not affected by ozone treatment, indicating a strong resistance to oxidation. These saturated and aliphatic carbons are

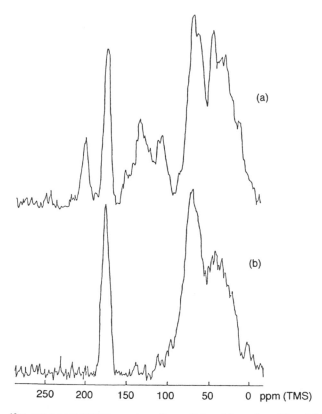

Figure 5.1. ^{13}C-CP-MAS NMR spectra of nondialyzable melanoidins (a) before and (b) after ozonolysis. Melanoidins were prepared from glucose and glycine at 95 °C and pH 6.8 for 7 h

supposed to form the skeleton or the backbone of melanoidins. Peaks III and IV which disappeared by ozone treatment are considered to be due to the cleavage of C=C and C=N bonds. These bonds are suggested to be important for the structure of the chromophores since the melanoidins were decolorized (to the extent of 97%) by ozonolysis (Kim *et al.*, 1985). In our previous studies (Kim *et al.*, 1985; Hayase *et al.*, 1984), we reported that furans and phenols were formed by hydrogen peroxide treatment but were not detected by ozone treatment. Accordingly, the contents of heterocyclic compounds in melanoidins are thought to be less abundant. Similar results were reported by Kato and Tsuchida (1981).

The ^{13}C NMR spectral data for Glc–Gly(2-^{13}C) MEL indicated that glycine is incorporated to a great extent into melanoidin molecules (Hayase *et al.*, 1986). Feather and Nelson (1984) reported similar results for Glc–Gly MEL and Fru–Gly MEL.

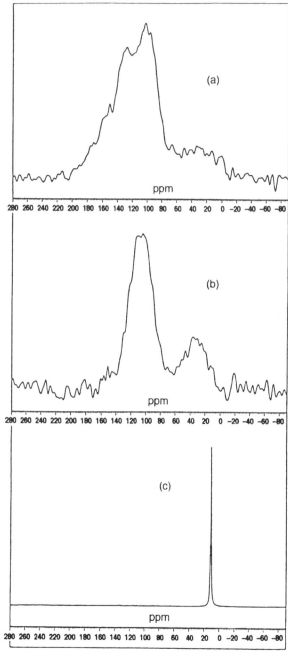

Figure 5.2. ^{15}N-CP-MAS NMR spectra of nondialyzable melanoidins prepared from the glucose–[15]N-glycine reaction system (a) before and (b) after ozonolysis, and ^{15}N-glycine

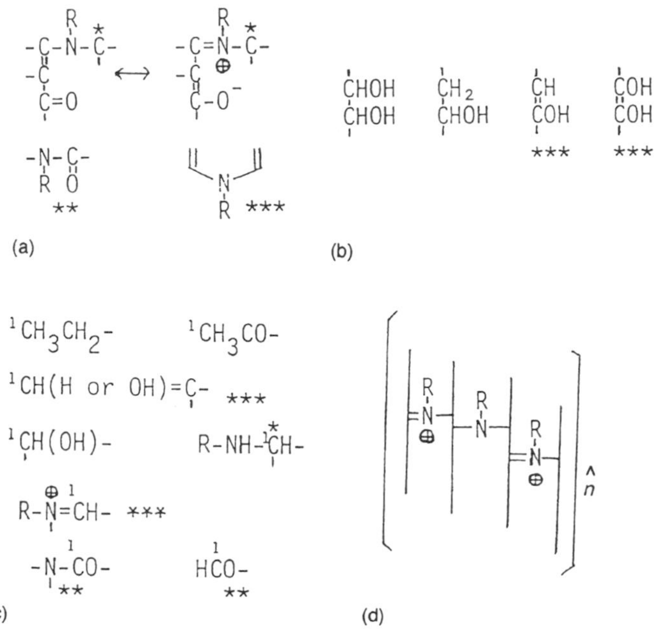

(a)

(b)

(c)

(d)

*   Carbons formed from amide after ozonolysis
** Minor structure
*** Carbons cleaved after ozonolysis
R=side chain of amino compounds

Figure 5.3. Proposed partial structure of melanoidins

Figure 5.2 shows the ^{15}N-CP-MAS NMR spectra of Glc–Gly (^{15}N) MEL, indicating a broad peak at 0–70 ppm (peak A), a large peak at 70–120 ppm (peak B) and a shoulder peak at 120–170 ppm (peak C). On ozonolysis, peak A was increased and peak C disappeared, as shown in Figure 5.2. Benzing-Purdie *et al.* (1983) reported that nitrogen in Xyl–Gly MEL was mainly in the secondary amide form. Although peaks around 100 ppm coincide closely with the chemical shift of amides (Levy and Lichter, 1978), the authors suggest that peak B is due to conjugated enamines (see Figure 5.3) and partly to amides. This suggestion is also supported by the ^{13}C NMR spectral data of Glc(1-^{13}C)– Gly MEL. Moreover, peak C is estimated to be mainly due to —C=N(+)< from the NMR spectra of ^{13}C-labeled melanoidins. Pyridine and pyrazine-type nitrogens are not present in the melanoidins, but the presence of pyrrole-type nitrogen is disputable.

Kato and Tsuchida (1981) have proposed a skeletal structure of Xyl– butylamine MEL from the data obtained by the thermal and oxidative

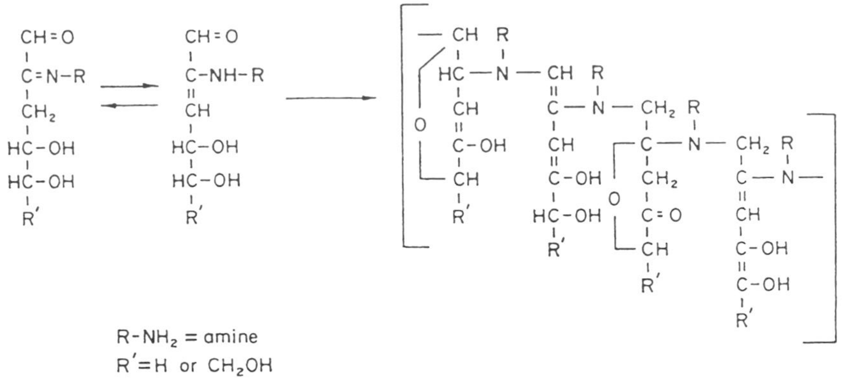

CH=O   CH=O   — CH   R
| | | |
C=N-R   ⟶   C-NH-R   ⟶   HC — N — CH   R
| ‖ | ‖ |
CH₂   CH   CH   C — N — CH₂ R
| | O | | | |
HC-OH   HC-OH   C-OH CH   C — N — CH₂ R
| | | ‖ | | | |
HC-OH   HC-OH   CH   C-OH CH₂ C — N —
| | | | O   ‖
R′   R′   R′   HC-OH C=O   CH
                                          | | |
                                          R′   CH   C-OH
                                                | ‖
                                                R′   C-OH
                                                     |
                                                     R′   ⌃
                                                              n

R-NH₂ = amine
R′=H or CH₂OH

Figure 5.4 Possible repeating units of melanoidins and their precursors. (Reprinted from Kato and Tsuchida, 1981, with kind permission from Elsevier Science Ltd)

decompositions, the number of hydroxyl groups (0.6–0.7 per Xyl moiety) in melanoidins and so on (Figure 5.4). The estimated structure principally supports the data from Motai (1976) which shows that melanoidins are chain polymers of homologous series bent symmetrically.

Figure 5.3 shows the partial chemical structure of melanoidins deduced from the above results.

DESMUTAGENIC EFFECTS OF MELANOIDINS

Melanoidins are known to have various functional properties, for example photosensitive effects (Gomyo and Miura, 1983), interaction with metal ions (Hashiba, 1986; Terasawa *et al.*, 1991), antioxidative effects (Kim *et al.*, 1986; Yamaguchi, 1986), antimicrobial action (Einarson and Eriksson, 1990), dietary fiber-like action (Gomyo and Miura, 1986), effect of enteric bacteria (Horikoshi *et al.*, 1981) and inhibition of trypsin (Hirano *et al.*, 1994). In this section, desmutagenic effects of melanoidins are reviewed.

Heterocyclic amines are formed by heating amino acids and proteins at high temperatures. In many cases these heterocyclic amines are mutagenic and carcinogenic. Glc–Gly MEL have strong desmutagenicity against their heterocyclic amines such as Trp–P-1 (3-amino-1, 4-dimethyl-5H-pyrido[4,3-b]indole, Trp–P-2 (3-amino-1-methyl-5H-pyrido[4,3-b]indole and Glu–P-1 (2-amino-6-methyldipyrido[1,2α:3′,2′-d]imidazole, as shown in Table 5.1 (Kim *et al.*, 1986; Kato *et al.*, 1985; Lee *et al.*, 1994). Melanoidins also showed (Table 5.1) a desmutagenic activity of 25–75% against mutagenic aromatic or heterocyclic compounds such as aflatoxin B₁, benzo[α]pyrene, 2-aminofluorene, 4-aminobiphenyl and 2-aminonaphthalene, as well as heterocyclic amines (Lee

Table 5.1. Desmutagenicity[a] of nondialyzable melanoidins (ND-MEL) and low molecular weight melanoidins (LM-MEL, MW = 500–1000) prepared from the glucose–glycine reaction system against mutagens

	Inhibition (%)[b]	
Mutagens	ND-MEL (2 mg/plate)	LM-MEL (4 mg/plate)
Trp–P-1	62.1	54.8
Trp–P-2	70.8	59.8
Glu–P-1	75.2	62.1
N–OH–Trp–P-2[c]	94.0	91.0

[a]Desmutagenicity against mutagens was assayed by the preincubation method (at 37 °C for 30 min) using *Salmonella typhimurium* TA98 in the presence of S9 mix. The mutagens were incubated with and without MEL at 37 °C for 30 min prior to preincubation.
[b]Inhibition (%) was calculated by the ratio of revertants/plate in $(+)/(-)$MEL.
[c]Synthesized 3-hydroxyamino-1-methyl-5H-pyrido[4,3-b]indole.

et al., 1994). The strong desmutagenic activity of melanoidins from various kinds of amino acids, peptides or egg albumin hydrolyzates with glucose was also found against Trp–P-1.

Heterocyclic amines have no mutagenicity without metabolic activation by cytochrome P-450 in hepatocyte (Yamazoe *et al.*, 1980). Figure 5.5 shows the mechanism of DNA damage by activation of heterocyclic amines, such as Trp–P-2. One pathway is considered to be initiated by hydroxylation of heterocyclic amines followed by acetylation and modification of guanine in DNA, resulting from the flame shift of DNA (Sugimura, 1982). However, the acetylation is not

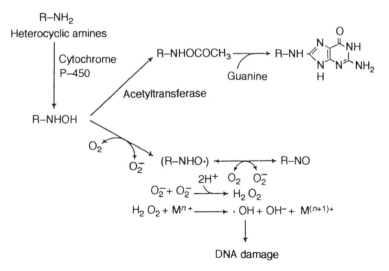

Figure 5.5. DNA damage by heterocyclic amines

necessary for the appearance of mutagenicity of Trp–P-1 and Trp–P-2 and so on (Nagao *et al.*, 1983). On the other hand, superoxides ($O_2^\bullet$) are formed by reduction of oxygen molecules by the oxidation of the NHOH form of heterocyclic amines (Nakayama *et al.* 1985). O_2 forms hydroxyl radicals ($^\bullet OH$) by disproportionation of $O_2^\bullet$ or Fenton's reaction, as shown in Figure 5.5. Hydroxyl radicals may damage DNA molecules.

Melanoidins were not affected by *Salmonella typhimurium* TA98 in the region of concentration used for the mutagenic test, the Ames test, and no effects on enzymatic activity in the S9 mix fraction of hepatic homogenates. Lee *et al.* (1994) observed desmutagenic activity greater than 90% against synthesized hydroxylamine derivatives, being the metabolically activated form of Trp–P-2. These findings suggest that desmutagenicity of melanoidins is due to the action against the hydroxylamine form of heterocyclic amines. Melanoidins are supposed to react directly with the NHOH group of the amines or scavenge the active oxygen species. It is expected that melanoidins show the desmutagenic activity *in vivo* in digestive organs because parts of melanoidins were absorbed through the gastrointestinal tract of rats (Lee *et al.*, 1992).

Melanoidins showed no desmutagenic activity against nitrosamines, which are mutagens and carcinogens produced by the nitrosation between nitriles and secondary amines in digestive organs and in processed foods. However, melanoidins inhibited the formation of nitrosamine by the reduction of nitrite as well as ascorbic acid because of a strong reducing ability (Kato *et al.*, 1987).

SCAVENGING OF HYDROXYL RADICALS BY MELANOIDINS

Figure 5.6 shows ESR spectra of DMPO (5,5-dimethyl-1-pyrroline-*N*-oxide) spin adduct formed by 10 kGy irradiation of Co-60 γ-rays in water. DMPO–OH showed quartet (1:2:2:1) signals because the hyperfine coupling constant of nitrogen is the same as that of hydrogen. DMPO–H split to triplet signals by the nitrogen atom followed by six to twelve signals by two hydrogen atoms with the same coupling constant, eventually resulting as nine signals (1:1:2:1:2:1:2:1:1), as shown in Figure 5.6.

When Glc–Gly MEL are added to water containing DMPO, the number of radicals was decreased by 10 kGy of γ-irradiation (Hayase *et al.*, 1989a, 1990). Mn^{2+} was used as an internal standard to calculate the relative amounts from ESR signal intensity. Melanoidins at a concentration of 0.3 or 0.03% scavenged 86 or 47% of hydroxyl radicals and 85 or 58% of H radicals. Although DMPO–OH is readily decomposed by reducing reagents, e.g. ascorbic acid, it was hardly decomposed by the addition of 0.3% melanoidins.

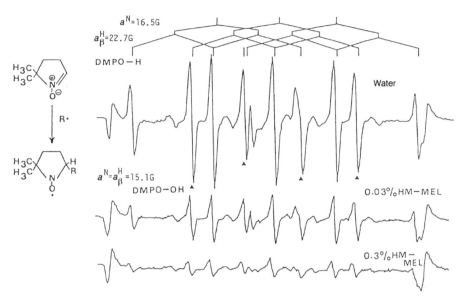

Figure 5.6. ESR spectra of DMPO–spin adducts formed by γ-irradiation (10 kGly) of water with or without nondialyzable melanoidins prepared from the glucose–glycine reaction system. (Reprinted with permission of Birkhäuser Verlag from Hayase *et al.*, 1990)

The authors also measured the effects of melanoidins on the ESR signal intensity of PBN (α-phenyl-*N-tert*-butylnitrone) spin adducts formed by γ-irradiation of 10 kGy compared with various scavengers (Table 5.2). The scavenging activity of hydroxyl radicals by low molecular weight melanoidins

Table 5.2. Effects of melanoidins prepared from the glucose–glycine reaction system on ESR signal intensity of PBN–OH spin adduct formed by γ-irradiation (10 kGly)

| | Scavenger concentration (%) | | |
Scavenger	0	0.2	0.5
ND-MEL	100	25	18
LM-MEL	100	44	19
R-MEL	100	63	24
Fructose	100	ND	80
Mannitol	100	ND	102
BSA	100	ND	68

ND-MEL = nondialyzable melanoidins.
LM-MEL = low molecular weight melanoidins (MW = 500–1000).
R-MEL = nondialyzable melanoidins reduced with $NaBH_4$.
BSA = bovine serum albumin.
ND = not determined.

(LM-MEL; MW = 500–1000) prepared from the glucose–glycine reaction system was rather weak compared with that by Glc–Gly MEL (HM-MEL; nondialyzable melanoidins). Scavenging activity of melanoidins on hydroxyl radicals was much higher than that of known scavengers of hydroxyl radicals such as fructose, mannitol and bovine serum albumin (BSA).

The higher scavenging rate of hydroxyl radicals by melanoidins may be due to their unique partial structure. It is difficult to characterize the partial structure of melanoidins, but the authors speculate that possible forms may be reductones, enamines or pyrrole-like structures (see the section on the chemical structure of melanoidins). Even when melanoidins were reduced with sodium borohydride, the scavenging activity of the reduced melanoidins (R-MEL) on hydroxyl radicals remained (Table 5.2).

Reductones in melanoidins are considered to be incompletely reduced by sodium borohydride, and enamine and pyrrole-like structures may be barely reduced. Moreover, melanoidins were reported to have relatively stable free radicals (Mitsuda *et al.*, 1965; Wu *et al.*, 1978). The free radicals are also supposed to be important for scavenging hydroxyl radicals.

SCAVENGING OF HYDROGEN PEROXIDES BY MELANOIDINS

Figure 5.7 shows the scavenging effects of melanoidins (HM-MEL and LM-MEL) on hydrogen peroxides at various concentrations. Hydrogen peroxides decreased with an increase in the concentration of melanoidins. The scavenging activity of HM-MEL was higher than that of LM-MEL (Hayase *et al.*, 1989, 1990). Kim *et al.* (1984) have reported that melanoidins were decolorized and decomposed by high concentrations of hydrogen peroxides. Such a reaction is considered to be mainly based on an attack on carbonyl groups of melanoidins by hydrogen peroxides. The reaction is supposed to be related to the scavenging action of hydrogen peroxides by melanoidins. Although melanoidins were decolorized up to approximately 21% by 10 kGy of γ-irradiation, they were not decomposed according to the results of measurements of mean molecular weight by gel permeation HPLC. Consequently, hydrogen peroxides generated by γ-irradiation may not degrade the main skeleton of melanoidins.

SCAVENGING OF SUPEROXIDES BY MELANOIDINS

Superoxides were measured by the increasing amount of the absorbance of 560 nm of diformazan formed by the reaction for 1 min after the addition of phenazine methosulfate (PMS) solution to NADPH and nitroblue tetrazonium (NBT) solutions by the method of Ponti *et al.* (1978). Superoxides are generated as described below:

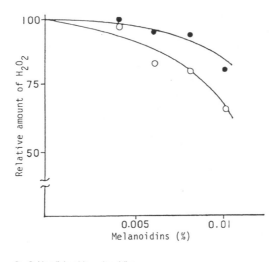

Figure 5.7. Scavenging of hydrogen peroxide by melanoidins prepared from the glucose–glycine reaction system. (Reprinted with permission of Birkhäuser Verlag from Hayase *et al.*, 1990)

$$NADPH + H^+ + PMS \longrightarrow NADPH^+ + PMSH_2$$
$$PMSH_2 + 2O_2 \longrightarrow 2O_2^- + 2H^+ + PMS$$
$$NBT + 2Cl^- + 4O_2^- + 4H^+ \longrightarrow diformazan + 4O_2 + 2HCl$$

Table 5.3 shows scavenging effects of melanoidins on superoxides. Melanoidins effectively scavenged superoxides to a similar degree to 16 units

Table 5.3. Effects of melanoidins prepared from the glucose–glycine reaction system on superoxide generated from the NADPH–PMS–NBT reaction system under aerobic conditions

Scavenger	Inhibition (%)
Control	0
ND-MEL (0.03%)	61
ND-MEL (0.06%)	74
LM-MEL (0.03%)	53
LM-MEL (0.06%)	71
Superoxide dismutase (16 units/ml)	83

ND-MEL = nondialyzable melanoidins.
LM-MEL = low molecular weight melanoidins (MW = 500–1000).

of superoxide dismutase (Hayase *et al.*, 1989; 1990). Scavenging activity of superoxides by HM-MEL was almost the same as that by LM-MEL.

Superoxides were reported to be scavenged by ascorbic acid which has reducing ability and antioxidative activity similar to melanoidins (Nishikimi, 1975; Cavelli and Bielski, 1983). The reaction rate constant $(5 \times 10^4 - 2.7 \times 10^5$ $M^{-1} s^{-1})$ of ascorbic acid against superoxides was markedly lower than that $(10^3 M^{-1} s^{-1})$ of superoxide dismutase (Nishikimi, 1975; Cavelli and Bielski, 1983). Accordingly, the scavenging ability of melanoidins on superoxides is much higher than that of ascorbic acid. These characteristics cannot be explained only by the reductone structure in melanoidins because the reducing ability of melanoidins is 0.71 as compared to the equivalent weight of ascorbic acid per weight of melanoidins (Kim *et al.*, 1986).

SCAVENGING OF ACTIVE OXYGENS BY GLYCATED PROTEINS

Proteins can react with reducing sugars to produce Amadori compounds, which are the products of the early stage, followed by modification into colored, fluorescent and crosslinked molecules in the last stage. The glycated proteins possess antioxidative activity on lipid peroxidation, although the activity is not as strong as that of melanoidins (Utsunomiya *et al.*, 1983). Therefore, the glycated proteins are also expected to have scavenging activity against active oxygen species.

Table 5.4 shows scavenging activities of hydroxyl radicals and hydrogen peroxides by glycated proteins and model compounds of Maillard reaction products. Glycated BSA at a concentration of 0.5% scavenged 34% of hydroxyl radicals, while BSA at a concentration of 0.5% scavenged 15% of hydroxyl radicals (Okamoto *et al.*, 1992). Amadori compounds, *N*-deoxyfructosylbutylamine, had no activity of scavenging of hydroxyl radicals. Pyrraline, which is known as one of the advanced Maillard reaction products (Nakayama *et al.*, 1980), was detected *in vivo* (Hayase *et al.*, 1989b; Miyata and Monnier, 1992), while caproyl pyrraline and BSA coupled with caproyl pyrraline had a significant activity against hydroxyl radicals. This indicates that the scavenging rate of hydroxyl radicals by glycated proteins may not be due to the Maillard reaction products in the early stage but to those in the advanced stage.

BSA, insulin and lysozyme incubated with glucose at 50 °C had a much stronger scavenging activity of hydrogen peroxides than untreated proteins (Table 5.4). Molecular weight and amino acid residues of BSA and glycated BSA treated with hydrogen peroxides did not change. Therefore, Maillard reaction products in glycated proteins but not the protein itself take part in their scavenging activities against hydrogen peroxides. *N*-Glucosylbutylamine

Table 5.4. The effects of Maillard reaction products on ESR signal intensity of DMPO–OH spin adduct formed by γ-irradiation (10 kGy) and scavenging of hydrogen peroxide

Scavenger	Relative ESR signal intensity	Scavenged H_2O_2 (nmol)
Control	100	0
BSA (0.5%)	85	—
BSA (0.036%)	—	0.36
G-BSA (0.5%)	66	—
G-BSA (0.036%)	—	4.11
GB (0.036%)	—	2.56
DB (0.036%)	—	4.47
DB (1.0%)	100	—
CP (0.036%)	—	0
CP (1.0%)	61	—
P-BSA (0.036%)	—	0.36
P-BSA (1.0%)	48	—

G-BSA = BSA incubated with glucose at 50 °C for 15 days.
GB = N-glucosylbutylamine.
DB = N-deoxyfructosylbutylamine.
CP = caproyl pyrraline.
P-BSA = bovine serum albumin coupled with CP.

and *N*-deoxyfructosylbutylamine had a strong scavenging activity toward hydrogen peroxides, while caproyl pyrraline and BSA coupled with caproyl pyrraline had little or no scavenging activity. The Maillard reaction products in an early stage are presumed to be involved in the scavenging activity of glycated proteins against hydrogen peroxide. These scavenging activities of glycated proteins on hydroxyl radicals and hydrogen peroxides are considered to be partly due to melanoidin-like pigments in glycated proteins, as described above.

On the other hand, glycated BSA had weaker scavenging activity than BSA against superoxides because of the formation of superoxides from glycated BSA. It has also been demonstrated that the superoxide radicals are generated by Amadori compounds (Azevedo *et al.*, 1988).

SUMMARY

Melanoidins demonstrate physiologically positive effects because of unique partial structures in the molecules such as reductones, enamines and pyrrole-like structures. Melanoidins have a strong scavenging activity against active oxygen species, e.g. hydroxyl radicals, hydrogen peroxides and superoxides. The scavenging of active oxygen species by melanoidins seems to be significant for the explanation of the appearance of the antioxidative and desmutagenic activities. Strong scavenging activity by glycated proteins toward hydrogen peroxides is presumed to be based on the Amadori compounds and melanoidins. Advanced Maillard products such as pyrraline and melanoidins may participate in the scavenging of hydroxyl radicals by glycated proteins.

ACKNOWLEDGMENTS

The author's studies were carried out together with Professor Hiromichi Kato at Ohtsuma University and many of his coworkers. The author wishes to thank Professor H. Kato and his coworkers for helpful discussions and for their expert work.

REFERENCES

Azevedo, M., Falcao, J., Paposo, J., and Manso, C. (1988). Superoxide radical generation by Amadori compounds, *Free Rad. Res. Commun.*, **4**, 331–5.

Benzing-Purdie, L. M., and Ratcliffe, C. I. (1986). A study of the Maillard reaction by ^{13}C and ^{15}N CP-MAS NMR: influence of time, temperature, and reactants on major products, *Dev. Food Sci.*, **13**, 193–206.

Benzing-Purdie, L. M., Ripmeester, J. A., and Preston, C. M. (1983). Elucidation of the nitrogen forms in melanoidins and humic acid by nitrogen-15 cross polarization-magic angle spinning nuclear magnetic resonance, *J. Agric. Food Chem.*, **31**, 913–15.

Benzing-Purdie, L. M., Cheshire, M. V., Williams, B. I., Sparling, G. P., Ratcliffe, C. I., and Ripmeester, J. A. (1986). Fate of [^{15}N] glycine in peat as determined by ^{13}C and ^{15}N CP-MAS NMR spectroscopy, *J. Agric. Food Chem.*, **34**, 170–6.

Cavelli, D. E., and Bielski, B. H. J. (1983). Kinetics and mechanism for the oxidation of ascorbic acid/ascorbate by HO_2/O_2^- radicals. A pulse radiolysis and stopped-flow photolysis study, *J. Phys. Chem.*, **87**, 1807–12.

Einarson, H., and Eriksson, C. (1990). The antibacterial effect of Maillard reaction products and sorbic acid at different pH levels and temperatures. In P. A. Finot, H. U. Aeschbacher, R. F. Hurrell and R. Liardon (eds.), *The Maillard Reaction in Food Processing, Human Nutrition and Physiology*, Birkhauser Verlag, Basel, pp. 227–32.

Feather, M. S., and Nelson, D. (1984) Maillard polymers derived from D-glucose, D-fructose, 5-(hydroxymethyl)-2-furaldehyde, and glycine and methionine, *J. Agric. Food Chem.*, **32**, 1428–32.

Gomyo, T., and Miura, M. (1983). Melanoidin in foods: chemical and physiological aspects, *J. Jap. Soc. Nutr. Food Sci.*, **36**, 331–40.

Gomyo, T., and Miura, M. (1986). Effect of melanoidin on the digestion and absorption of disaccharides in the small intestine of rats, *Dev. Food Sci.*, **13**, 549–58.

Hashiba, H. (1986). Oxidative browning of Amadori compounds—color formation by iron with Maillard reaction products, *Dev. Food Sci.*, **13**, 155–64.

Hayase, F., and Kato, H. (1985). Maillard reaction products from D-glucose and butylamine, *Agric. Biol. Chem.*, **49**, 467–73.

Hayase, F., and Kato, H. (1986). Low-molecular Maillard reaction products and their formation mechanisms, *Dev. Food Sci.*, **13**, 39–48.

Hayase, F., and Kato, H. (1994). Maillard reaction products: safety and physiologic effects, *Comments Agric. Food Chem.*, **3**, 111–28.

Hayase, F., Kim, S. B., and Kato, H. (1984). Decolorization and degradation products of the melanoidins by hydrogen peroxide, *Agric. Biol. Chem.*, **48**, 2711–17.

Hayase, F., Kim, S. B., and Kato, H. (1986). Analyses of the chemical structures of melanoidins by ^{13}C NMR, ^{13}C and ^{15}N CP-MAS spectrometry, *Agric. Biol. Chem.*, **50**, 1951–7.

Hayase, F., Hirashima, S., Okamoto, G., and Kato, H. (1989a). Scavenging of active oxygens by melanoidins, *Agric. Biol. Chem.*, **53**, 3383–5.

Hayase, F., Nagaraj, R. H., Miyata, S., Njoroge, F. G., and Monnier, V. M. (1989b). Aging of proteins: immunological detection of a glucose-derived pyrrole formed during Maillard reaction *in vivo, J. Biol. Chem.*, **264**, 3758–64.

Hayase, F., Hirashima, S., Okamoto, G. and Kato, H. (1990). Scavenging of active oxygens by melanoidin. In P. A. Finot, H. U. Aeschbacher, R. F. Hurrell, and R. Liardon (eds.), *The Maillard Reaction in Food Processing, Human Nutrition and Physiology*, Birkhäuser Verlag, Basel, pp. 361–6.

Hayashi, T., and Namiki, M. (1986a). Role of sugar fragmentation in the Maillard reaction, *Dev. Food Sci.*, **13**, 29–38.

Hayashi, T., and Namiki, M. (1986b). Role of sugar fragmentation in an early stage browning of amino-carbonyl reaction of sugar with amino acids, *Agric. Biol. Chem.*, **50**, 1965–70.

Hirano, M., Miura, M., and Gomyo, T. (1994). Melanoidin as a novel trypsin inhibitor, *Biosci. Biotechnol. Biochem.*, **58**, 940–1.

Homma, S., Tomura, T., and Fujimaki, M. (1982). Fractionation of nondialyzable melanoidin into components by electrofocusing electrophoresis, *Agric. Biol. Chem.*, **46**, 1791–6.

Horikoshi, M., Ohmura, M., Gomyo, T., Kuwabara, Y., and Ueda, S. (1981). Effects of browning products on the intestinal microflora of the rat, *Prog. Food Nutr. Sci.*, **5**, 223–8.

Ikan, R., Dorsey, T., and Kaplan, I. R. (1990). Characterization of natural and synthetic humic substances (melanoidins) by stable carbon and nitrogen isotope measurements and elemental compositions, *Anal. Chim. Acta.*, **232**, 11–18.

Kato, H., and Tsuchida, H. (1981). Estimation of melanoidin structure by pyrolysis and oxidation, *Prog. Food Nutr. Sci.*, **5**, 147–56.

Kato, H., Kim, S. B., Hayase, F., and Chuyen, N. V. (1985). Desmutagenicity of melanoidins against mutagenic pyrolysates, *Agric. Biol. Chem.*, **49**, 3093–5.

Kato, H., Lee, I. E., Chuyen, N. V., Kim, S. B., and Hayase, F. (1987). Inhibition of nitrosamine formation by nondialyzable melanoidins, *Agric. Biol. Chem.*, **51**, 1333–8.

Kim, S. B., Hayase, F., and Kato, H. (1985). Decolorization and degradation products of melanoidins on ozonolysis, *Agric. Biol. Chem.*, **49**, 785–792.

Kim, S. B., Hayase, F., and Kato, H. (1986). Desmutagenic effects of melanoidins against amino acid and protein pyrolyzates, *Dev. Food Sci.*, **13**, 383–92.

Lee, I. E., Chuyen, N. V., Hayase, F., and Kato, H. (1992). Absorption and distribution of [^{14}C]-melanoidins in rats and the desmutagenicity of absorbed melanoidins against Trp–P-1, *Biosci. Biotechnol. Biochem.*, **56**, 21–3.

Lee, I. E., Chuyen, N. V., Hayase, F., and Kato, H. (1994). Desmutagenicity of melanoidins against various kinds of mutagens and activated mutagens, *Biosci. Biotechnol. Biochem.*, **58**, 18–23.

Levy, G. C., and Lichter, R. (1978). *Nitrogen-15 Nuclear Magnetic Resonance Spectroscopy*, John Wiley & Sons, New York, p. 28.

Mitsuda, H., Yasumoto, K., and Yokoyama, K. (1965). Studies on the free radical in amino-carbonyl reaction. *Agric. Biol. Chem.*, **29**, 751–6.

Miyata, S., and Monnier, V. M. (1992). Immunohistochemical detection of advanced glycosylation end products in diabetic tissues using monoclonal antibody to pyrraline, *J. Clin. Invest.*, **89**, 1102–12.

Motai, H. (1976). Viscosity of melanoidins formed by oxidative browning: validity of the equation for a relationship between color intensity and molecular weight of melanoidin, *Agric. Biol. Chem.*, **40**, 1–7.

Nagao, M., Fujita, Y., Wakabayashi, K., and Sugimura, T. (1983). Ultimate forms of mutagenic and carcinogenic heterocyclic amines produced by pyrolysis, *Biochem. Biophys. Res. Commun.*, **114**, 626–31.

Nakayama, T., Hayase, F., and Kato, H. (1980). Formation of ε-(2-formyl-5-hydroxymethyl-pyrrol-1-yl)-L-norleucine in the Maillard reaction between D-glucose and L-lysine, *Agric. Biol. Chem.*, **44**, 1201–2.

Nakayama, T., Kaneko, M., Kodama, M., and Nagata, C. (1985). Cigarette smoke induces single strand breaks of DNA in human cells, *Nature*, **314**, 462–4.

Namiki, M. (1988). Chemistry of Maillard reaction: recent studies on the browning reaction mechanism and the development of antioxidants and mutagens, *Adv. Food Res.*, **32**, 115–84.

Nishikimi, M. (1975). Oxidation of ascorbic acid with superoxide anion generated by the xanthine–xanthine oxidase system, *Biochem. Biophys. Res. Commun.*, **63**, 463–8.

Okamoto, G., Hayase, F., and Kato, H. (1992). Scavenging of active oxygen species by glycated proteins, *Biosci. Biotechnol. Biochem.*, **56**, 928–31.

Piattell, M. (1961). The structure of melanins and melanogenesis-I. The structure of melanin in SEPIA, *Tetrahedron*, **15**, 66–75.

Ponti, V., Dianzani, M. U., Cheeseman, K., and Slater, T. F. (1978). Studies on the reduction of nitroblue tetrazolium chloride mediated through the action of NADH and phenazine methosulphate, *Chem. Biol. Interact.*, **23**, 281–91.

O'Reilly, R. (1983). Application of electrofocusing for the fractionation of colored products formed during the xylose–glycine Maillard reaction, *Chem. Ind.*, **19**, 716–17.

Sugimura, T. (1982). Mutagens in cooked food. In R. A. Fleck and A. Hollaender (eds.), *Genetic Toxicology*, Plenum Publishers, New York, pp. 243–69.

Terasawa, N., Murata, M., and Homma, S. (1991). Separation of model melanoidin into components with copper chelating Sepharose 6B column chromatography and comparison of chelating activity, *Agric. Biol. Chem.*, **55**, 1507–14.

Utsunomiya, N., Hayase, F., and Kato, H. (1983). Antioxidative activities of Maillard reaction products of D-glucose with ovalbumin hydrolyzed by proteases, and their synergistic effect with tocopherols, *J. Jap. Soc. Nutr. Food Sci.*, **36**, 461–5.

Wu, C. H., Russell, G., and Powrie, W. D. (1987). Paramagnetic behavior of model system melanoidins, *J. Food Sci.*, **52**, 813–22.

Yamaguchi, N. (1986). Antioxidative activity of the oxidation products prepared from melanoidins, *Dev. Food Sci.*, **13**, 291–9.

Yamazoe, Y., Ishii, K., Kamataki, T., Kato, R., and Sugimura, T. (1980). Isolation and characterization of active metabolisms of tryptophan–pyrolysate mutagen, TRP-P-2, formed by rat liver microsomes, *Chem. Biol. Interact.*, **30**, 125–38.

6

The Impact of the Maillard Reaction on the Nutritional Value of Food Proteins

MENDEL FRIEDMAN

USDA-ARS, Western Regional Research Center, Albany, California, USA

INTRODUCTION

Amino–carbonyl and related interactions of food constituents encompass those changes commonly termed 'browning' reactions. Specifically, reactions of amines, amino acids, peptides and proteins with reducing sugars and vitamin C (nonenzymatic browning) and quinones (enzymatic browning) cause deterioration of food during storage and commercial or domestic processing. The loss of nutritional quality is attributed to the destruction of essential amino acids and a decrease in digestibility. The production of antinutritional and toxic compounds may further reduce the nutritional value and possibly the safety of foods.

Such Maillard reactions occur widely in foods subjected to heat processing and storage. The chemical nature of the transformation of the initial stages of the Maillard reactions involves the formation of a Schiff's base (aldamine) between the amino and carbonyl group. This is followed by the rearrangement of the Schiff's base to an Amadori compound (1-amino-1-deoxy-2-ketose). The Amadori compounds then react further by several pathways, including enolization, dehydration, aldol condensations and Strecker degradation, to form a large number of compounds. Although extensive efforts have been made to elucidate the chemistry of both desirable and undesirable

The Maillard Reaction: Consequences for the Chemical and Life Sciences. Edited by Raphael Ikan
©1996 John Wiley & Sons Ltd

compositional changes during browning, parallel studies on the nutritional and toxicological consequences of browning are limited. Reported studies in this area include (a) influence of damage to essential amino acids, especially arginine, lysine, methionine and tryptophan, on nutritional quality; (b) attempts to restore nutritional quality by fortifying browning products with essential amino acids; (c) nutritional damage as a function of processing conditions; (d) biological utilization and metabolism of characterized browning product; (e) formation of food toxicants including kidney-damaging compounds, growth inhibitors, mutagenic (DNA-damaging), clastogenic (chromosome-damaging) and carcinogenic compounds; and (f) formation of beneficial compounds including antioxidants and anticarcinogens.

In order to develop rational approaches to minimize adverse consequences of Maillard reactions and optimize beneficial ones, studies are needed to relate compositional changes to nutritional and toxicological consequences. To catalyze progress, a need exists to define known chemical, biochemical, nutritional and toxicological indices or parameters of nonenzymatic browning and its prevention. This review addresses only the nutritional consequences of the Maillard reaction from selected studies in the widely scattered literature. Specifically covered are the following aspects of the Maillard reaction: (a) *in vitro* and *in vivo* methods used to assess protein nutrition; (b) the nutritional value of glycated proteins and Maillard reaction products; and (c) possible approaches to prevent food browning.

Browning may also create desirable food attributes such as improved storage, flavor, color and the formation of antioxidants and antibacterial compounds. These aspects are beyond the scope of this review.

NUTRITIONAL PARAMETERS

AMINO ACID ANALYSIS

A key element of any nutritional evaluation of a food protein is its amino acid composition. Automated procedures are now widely used to achieve this objective. In developing such a procedure, Cavins and Friedman[1] recommended that the results should be presented in several forms, suitable for a variety of needs, as illustrated in Table 6.1. The nitrogen recovery parameter gives a check on the analysis. The ratio of amino acids is especially useful in highlighting decreases in specific amino acids, such as lysine, following physical or chemical modifications of proteins during food processing.

Sarwar *et al.*[2] described inter- and intralaboratory variations in amino acid composition of several protein sources: casein, soy protein, pea flour, whole wheat flour, egg white solids, minced beef and rapeseed concentrate. The interlaboratory measurements of isoleucine, leucine, lysine, phenylalanine, threonine and valine (coefficient of variation, CV, $<10\%$) were generally less

Table 6.1. Typical amino acid analysis parameters listed on a computer-generated printout. (Adapted from Ref. 1)

Sample parameters	Computer calculated values
N (%) (Kjeldahl)	mmoles/100 g sample
Protein (%) (N × 6.25)	g/100 g sample
Weight of sample (mg)	g/g N
Weight of N (mg)	g/16 g N
Method of hydrolysis, e.g. sealed tube	% N recovered
mg N/mL	% sample weight as amino acids
mg sample/mL	Mole %
Humin (%)	Weight %
	Ratios of each amino acid to all others

variable than those of tryptophan (CV of 14–20%) and cystine and methionine (CV of 10–17%). Variation between duplicate hydrolysates within laboratories was smaller than that between laboratories.

Possible variations in amino acid composition of the same protein sources should be taken into account when using these data to calculate nutritional parameters of foods.

AVAILABLE LYSINE

Chemically available or 'reactive' lysine content of a protein may be defined as the concentration of lysine ε-NH_2 groups that were unaffected during exposure of the protein to a sugar or other compound. The difference between total lysine (or lysine content before reaction) and available lysine indicates the number of lysine sites that have been chemically altered. Although standard amino acid analysis techniques can be used to estimate the total lysine content of a protein, this is not the case for available lysine, since, for example, labile Schiff's bases and isopeptide bonds between ε-NH_2 and COOH groups do not survive acid conditions used for protein hydrolysis. The lysine content of a browned product measured by amino acid analysis is sometimes higher than is actually the case. Acid hydrolysis of labile Schiff's bases and isopeptide bonds liberates free lysine so that the determined lysine value is higher than either what was actually present originally or what is nutritionally available. For example, Friedman[3] found that exposure of casein or soy protein to heat in the presence of glucose induced variable losses in lysine depending on the severity of treatment (Table 6.2). However, the listed values may not reflect the real situation (Figure 6.1). (The data also show that the severe treatments also induced a significant decrease in the arginine content of the proteins.) For the reasons given, extensive efforts have been made to determine chemically

Table 6.2. Lysine and arginine content of casein and soybean proteins treated with glucose. (Adapted from Ref. 3)

Amino acid	Casein control	Casein + 10% glucose (37 °C, 10 d)[a]	Casein + 10% glucose (95 °C, 4 h)[b]	Soy protein control	Soy protein + 10% glucose (37 °C, 10 d)[a]	Soy protein + 10% glucose (95 °C, 10 d)[b]
Lys	6.74[c]	5.68	3.47	5.67	4.15	2.66
Arg	2.73	2.62	0.88	5.74	5.50	2.51

[a]Mild browning.
[b]Severe browning.
[c]Values in mole %.

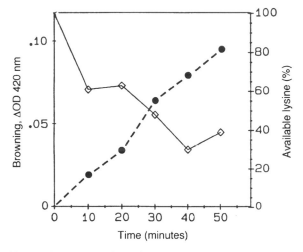

Figure 6.1 Effect on browning of heating soybean Kunitz trypsin inhibitor plus glucose at 120 °C and content of available lysine[79]

reactive or available lysine as an assessment of nutritionally bioavailable or biologically utilizable lysine. These studies are critically examined elsewhere.[4–7]

One such simple, rapid and inexpensive method is a modified ninhydrin assay for the measurement of available lysine.[8–10] The assay is based on the fact that amino groups react with ninhydrin to form a colored chromophore. The assay works well for pure proteins but is less effective for cereal grains, due probably to the inability of the ninhydrin solution to completely solubilize proteins such as glutenin and gliadin in a complex carbohydrate matrix. Our studies have developed an improved lithium acetate–dimethyl sulfoxide ninhydrin reagent.[9] This new reagent (a) diffuses into complex food matrices; (b) rapidly extracts the proteins; (c) increases the rate of reaction; and (d) stabilizes the ninhydrin chromophore. This method works well for proteins, grain flours, legumes and dairy products.

DIGESTIBILITY

Oste *et al.*[11] carried out elegant double-isotope studies in an effort to define possible effects of Maillard products on protein digestion. They found that a number of low molecular weight compounds from a glucose–lysine reaction mixture reduced plasma levels of dietary protein-derived lysine. The pure compounds also inhibited *in vitro* the enzymes aminopeptidase and carboxy-peptidase. They conclude that although the concentrations of furane, heterocyclic Maillard reaction products and fructosyl–lysine may be low, the combined effects of all of them on digestive enzymes may adversely affect dietary protein utilization.

Percival and Schneeman[12] examined long-term pancreatic response to feeding heat-damaged casein. They fed rats casein autoclaved at 121 °C for 24 hours. After 10 days, pancreatic amylase and chymotryptic activities were decreased, suggesting that turnover of the digestive enzymes is reduced when heat-damaged protein is fed. As a consequence, heat-damaged proteins are not digested and absorbed as well as unheated ones. The decreased pancreatic secretions contribute to the poor nutritional value of heated proteins.

In related studies, Friedman *et al.*[13–18] showed that kidney-damaging synthetic lysinoalanine[19] was a more effective inhibitor of carboxypeptidase than was ethylenediaminetetraacetic acid (EDTA). The enzyme was also inhibited by alkali-treated lysinoalanine containing food proteins such as casein, high-lysine corn protein, lactalbumin, soy protein and wheat gluten, and by the alkali-treated corn protein zein, which contained no lysinoalanine. Molecular mechanisms involving lysinoalanine formation, racemization, zinc chelation and protein unfolding were proposed to account for the inhibition of the zinc-containing carboxypeptidase. The inhibition could account in part for the reduced nutritional value of the alkali- and heat-treated proteins. Note that such treatments were carried out in the absence of carbohydrates.

Maillard products and glycated proteins impair digestibility by directly inhibiting digestive enzymes and/or blocking access of the enzymes to peptide bonds as a result of heat-induced chemical modification of the proteins by carbohydrates.

METHODS FOR EVALUATIN PROTEIN NUTRITIONAL VALUE

A large number of methods have been used to measure biological value, nutritional value or protein quality.[20] The labels of many foods now list the amount but not the quality of protein in the formulation. Because of large variations in the nutritional values of native and processed proteins derived from different sources,[21] it is important that the label give at least an indication of the quality of the protein. For example, although we may know the nutritional value of wheat gluten as a pure protein, its quality often deteriorates when wheat flour is processed into bread or cereals. Determining protein quality is important since it affects the entire world population, which must consume processed protein to survive. Industry has resisted adopting the widely used protein efficiency ratio (PER) method for measuring protein quality based on rat feeding studies because (a) it takes 28 days to complete; (b) it may be unreliable for some low-quality foods; (c) it may not be directly relevant to human nutrition; and (d) it may be too expensive when applied to food batches during the production process.

The following brief definitions outline the techniques mentioned in this paper:

Amino acid availability, % = (the total intake of amino acid minus the fecal excretion × 100)/(the total intake of amino acid)

Digestibility of nitrogen = [N intake — fecal N) × 100]/N intake

Limiting amino acid = an essential amino acid (lysine, methionine, threonine, tryptophan) in a protein that shows the greatest difference in concentration from the same amino acid in a reference, high-quality protein such as egg protein

Net protein ratio (NPR) = (weight gain of test animals + weight loss of animals fed non-protein basal diet)/(weight of protein consumed)

Net protein utilization (NPU) = (nitrogen retained/nitrogen intake) × 100

Protein efficiency ratio (PER) = (weight gain of a test group)/total protein consumed); C-PER = PER calculated from amino acid composition

Reference protein = a protein of high nutritional value containing an ideal pattern of amino acids

Generally, a PER below 1.5 approximately describes a low- or poor-quality protein; between 1.5 and 2.0, an intermediate quality; and above 2.0, a good to high quality.

NUTRITIONAL VALUE OF HEATED PROTEIN–CARBOHYDRATE MIXTURES

With this background, let us now examine some experimental findings on the nutritional and physiological aspects of consuming glycated proteins and characterized Maillard products.

CASEIN

Gumbmann *et al.*[22] and Smith and Friedman[23] evaluated the nutritional value and digestibilities of heat-damaged casein, casein–glucose and dry casein–starch mixtures (Table 6.3). The table shows the results for weight gain, digestibilities and PER. For samples held at 37 °C for 10 days, PER values tended to be somewhat lower than for the casein control. At 120 °C for 1 hour, PER of casein with added carbohydrates was slightly better than casein alone. Heating the samples at 180 °C reduced the PER below that of casein control, from 3.15 to 2.50 and to about 2 for the mixtures.

Heating at 240 °C for 1 hour reduced PER below a level that would support growth, with severe weight loss in rats. These negative PER values indicated a high degree of damage which occurred in casein, even in the absence of added glucose or starch. Heating at 240 °C reduced digestibilities to the minimum, which would result if the protein and carbohydrate were completely undigested. The lowest nitrogen digestibilities were found for the casein–glucose samples.

Table 6.3. Weight gain, PER and digestibilities of rats fed heat-damaged casein and casein-carbohydrate mixtures. (Adapted from Refs. 23 and 24)

Protein source	Weight gain (g)	PER	Nitrogen digestibility (%)
	37 °C for 10 days		
Casein control (unheated)	102	3.22	93.7
Casein	107	3.16	93.6
Casein + glucose	101	3.11	
Casein + starch	106	3.04	93.2
	120 °C for 1 hour		
Casein	99	3.08	93.1
Casein + glucose	116	3.37	93.4
Casein + starch	121	3.23	93.8
	180 °C for 1 hour		
Casein	63	2.50	72.9
Casein + glucose	41	1.86	84.6
Casein + starch	49	2.09	
	240 °C for 1 hour		
Casein	−17	−2.72	15.2
Casein + glucose	−17	−2.42	6.9
Casein + starch	−16	−2.54	14.9

Amino acid analysis of the treated samples revealed that there was no effect on amino acid composition at the 37 or 120 °C treatments. At 180 °C, there were no significant losses in amino acids for casein or casein plus glucose. At 240 °C, total amino acid concentration decreased from 25 to 45% for all samples and five new unidentified ninhydrin-positive peaks appeared on ion-exchange chromatograms. The most severely affected amino acids were, in decreasing order: threonine, serine, arginine, histidine, lysine, asparagine, isoleucine, glutamine and leucine. The low nitrogen digestion observed at 240 °C was not explained by conversion of even 50% of the amino acids into nondigestible compounds. In addition to the formation of these compounds, a portion of the remaining amino acids were also undigestible, and thus nutritionally unavailable.

This study shows that loss of nutritional quality of heat-treated casein, casein–glucose and casein–starch can be related to decreased nitrogen digestibilities as opposed to just destruction of essential amino acids. These changes impair intestinal absorption and nutritional quality in general. The possible formation of toxic compounds might also impair nutritional quality.

Chuyen *et al.*[24] examined nutritional and physiological effects of casein modified by glucose at 50 °C and 75% relative humidity for 1, 7 and 14 days and at 95 °C in aqueous solution. They report that (a) weight gain of rats fed the heated caseins decreased with the extent of modification; (b) biochemical parameters such as hematocrit, erythrocyte, leucocyte, GOT, GPT, triglycerides and cholesterol in serum were not affected by the treatments; (c) serum glucose levels of rats fed the browned caseins were significantly lower than those of unheated controls; and (c) supplementation of the heated samples with amino acids lost during the Maillard reactions did not restore the nutritional quality. These findings suggest that the heat treatments also induced the formation of antinutritional compounds which adversely affected protein quality.

Based on the utilization by rats of ^{14}C-labeled casein browned with glucose at 37 °C, Mori and Nakatsuji[25] concluded that the main reason for the observed reduction in nutritive value may be the reduction in absorption from the intestine of browning-induced lysine derivatives.

Evangelisti *et al.*[26] found that the amount of lysine blocked as lactuloselysine in milk formulae increased with the lactose protein ratio up to 20%. Partial substitution of lactose with dextrin resulted in a decrease in blocked lysine. However, addition of glucose enhanced the amount of blocked lysine measured as furosine.

Feeding casein and cod fish proteins sterilized in an autoclave at 121 °C in the presence of glucose resulted in lower digestibility and growth in rats compared to the unheated proteins.[27] The authors suggest that urinary taurine may serve as an indicator of nutritional damage for food proteins with inadequate sulfur amino acid content.

COMPARISON OF CASEIN AND LACTALBUMIN

Keyes *et al.*[28] studied the effects of autoclaving at 121 °C for 30 and 90 min in the presence of lactose on the protein quality of casein and lactalbumin. They found that the PER of casein was less susceptible to damage than that of lactalbumin and that the available lysine (but not total lysine) correlated with protein quality as measured by PER. This finding suggests that casein rather than lactalbumin (which may have contained small amounts of lactose) may be a better reference protein than lactalbumin for studies of nutritional value of foods and feeds. Washing of lactalbumin to remove any lactose present may alleviate or avoid this problem.

These authors also suggest the use of the so-called modified PER which avoids the problems that (a) the standard PER underestimates protein quality of lower quality proteins because it does not measure protein needs for maintenance and (b) the NPR and NPU methods overestimate protein quality because rats conserve protein when fed a nonprotein diet.

EGG PROTEINS

Tanaka *et al.*[29] and Lee *et al.*[30] carried out long-term studies on the nutritional and toxicological effects of nonenzymatic Maillard browning of egg albumin. Egg albumin and D-glucose were mixed in a ratio of 3 : 2. Water was added to give a moisture content of 15%. The mixture was then stored as 37 °C for 10 days. The brown product was freeze-dried and incorporated in dietary formulations.

The PER value of the control egg albumin decreased from 3.0 to 1.1 after browning. Long-term feeding studies revealed that rats on brown and control diets (5% egg albumin + 5% nonessential amino acids, PER = 1.1) gained weight equally for the first month. Those on the browned diet then began to lag behind the control diet group even though the PER values of both diets were the same. After 3 months, rats on brown diets weighed 30% less than those on the control diet. This difference after 6 or 12 months was about 25%. These results show that the rats did not adapt themselves to the brown diet over the one-year feeding period and that other factors associated with the brown diet affected nutritional quality.

These factors could be the formation of toxic compounds during browning. This suggestion is reinforced by the observation that rats fed brown diets had enlarged organs (hearts, livers, kidneys and spleens). This was accompanied by increased activities of liver enzymes in the serum, suggesting adverse effects on liver function. Also black–brown pigments of an unknown nature were found in the liver. The observed higher serum glucose levels with the brown diets also suggests physiological stress. Male rats were more susceptible than females to the brown-diet-induced physiological and toxicological stress (cf. Ref. 31). The authors concluded that browned proteins may induce damaging physiological and toxicological effects that are not detectable by chemical or short-term nutritional studies.

Kato et al.[32,33] compared the relative potencies of glucose and lactose on browning of ovalbumin, which they isolated from fresh egg whites. They found that (a) the free amino groups in ovalbumin–glucose and ovalbumin–lactose decreased, respectively, to 20 and 26% of the original values after storage for 26 days at 50 °C; (b) browning of ovalbumin–glucose was rapid, whereas that of ovalbumin–lactose was not significant; (c) removal of unreacted free glucose from the ovalbumin–glucose mixture strongly suppressed browning; (d) browning resumed when glucose was re-added; (e) addition of lactose to ovalbumin–glucose had a minor effect on browning; (f) SDS–polyacrylamide gel electrophoretic studies revealed that glucose also strongly accelerated protein polymerization.

The authors suggested that the accelerated polymerization of the glucose system might be due to degradation of fructosyllysine into reactive intermediates which induce polymerization, possibly through crosslinking. This suggestion is supported by a proposed mechanism of browning induced by glucose and lactose, respectively, which predicts a protective effect of 4-*O*-methyl-D-glucose against browning. This prediction was confirmed experimentally.

These observations showed that reducing monosaccharides such as glucose or galactose behaved differently in the browning reactions than disaccharides such as lactose. Possible nutritional consequences of such differences await more detailed study.

COMPARISON OF CASEIN, SOYBEAN AND EGG PROTEINS

A key question in assessing the nutritional value of heated protein–carbohydrate mixtures is the relative susceptibility of different proteins to different carbohydrates. To address this issue, Knipfel et al.[34] investigated the effects of carbohydrate–heat interactions on the nutritive value of casein, soy and egg proteins. They fed rats proteins that were autoclaved in the presence of 10% carbohydrates for various time periods. The following is a brief summary of this important study: (a) weight gain and food intake of rats fed egg protein were reduced more rapidly by autoclaving, regardless of carbohydrate present, than were those of casein and soy fed rats; (b) NPR of egg protein rapidly decreased with heating to the same value as soy, while casein was more resistant to protein damage; (c) digestibility of egg protein was reduced more severely than that of casein or soy protein; and (d) the presence of glucose, fructose or sucrose during autoclaving of the proteins reduced nutritive value more than autoclaving the pure proteins alone, while starch or cellulose had little effect on nutritional quality. These results show that egg protein was much more susceptible to damage than casein or soy proteins.

Lysine is the first limiting amino acid in egg protein and methionine/cystine in casein and soy protein. Proteins with lysine as the first limiting amino acid such as in egg and wheat proteins may be more susceptible to reduction in availability as a result of heating than is methionine. The results also show that reducing sugars such as glucose are more damaging to nutritive value than the nonreducing polysaccharides cellulose and starch.

COMPARISON OF COTTONSEED, PEANUT AND SOYBEAN PROTEINS

Rhee and Rhee[35] evaluated the effect on protein quality of mixing defatted flours and protein isolates from cottonseed, peanut and soybeans with glucose or sucrose in a ratio of 1 : 1 by weight followed by heating at 100 °C for 0, 2 or 6 hours. They reported that (a) sucrose-complexed proteins changed very little in *in vitro* digestibilities, available lysine, total amino acids and computed PER (C-PER) (b) the glucose complexes decreased substantially in the quality indexes mentioned; (c) lysine-rich soy protein lost a greater percent of its lysine than lysine-poor peanut and cottonseed proteins; and (d) protein digestibility, available lysine and C-PER were all highly correlated with a browning index, and available lysine was highly correlated with C-PER. Heat is widely used to inactivate antinutritional trypsin inhibitors in legumes.[36]

POTATO BROWNING

Sugars and starch exist together in potato tubers. They undergo continual enzyme-catalyzed transformations as shown in the following schematic:

$$\text{SUCROSE} \leftrightarrows \text{GLUCOSE} + \text{FRUCTOSE}$$
$$\uparrow\downarrow$$
$$\text{STARCH} \leftrightarrows \text{GLUCOSE}$$

Above 10 °C, the sugars and starch remain in balance, with the sugars either reforming into starch or being used up in the reactions. Below 10 °C, however, reducing sugars start to accumulate. Low-temperature storage may be undesirable because they can participate in Maillard reactions during processing.[37,38]

Although Maillard reactions in potatoes may cause some nutritional damage to potatoes, they induce the formation of brown colors in fried potatoes which some consumers prefer. Marquez and Anon[39] reported that both free amino acids and sugars participated in color development of potatoes during frying, with the amount of reducing sugar being the limiting parameter. Fructose caused the highest browning followed by glucose, whereas addition of sucrose caused minor color changes. The temperature dependence of color formation at low reducing sugar levels followed first-order kinetics with an activation energy (E_a) of 31 kcal/mole.

Enzymatic browning of potatoes also deserves comment. Chlorogenic acid (5-*O*-caffeoylquinic acid) constitutes up to about 90% of the total polyphenolic content of potatoes. The compound may be responsible for the bluish-gray coloration of boiled or steamed potatoes following exposure to air and for enzymatic browning.[40] It may also be involved in defenses of the potato plant against insect and phytopathogens. It affects the taste of the potato, is a strong antioxidant and is reported to inhibit phorbol-ester-induced skin tumor promotion. As part of an effort to improve the quality and safety of potatoes, we measured effects of light and food processing conditions on the chlorogenic acid content of potatoes and weed seeds.[41-43] Exposure to fluorescent light increased the chlorogenic acid content of tubers. Oven-baked potatoes contained 0% of the original amount of chlorogenic acid, boiled potatoes 35% and microwaved potatoes 55%. Commercially processed french fries, mashed potato flakes and potato skins contained no chlorogenic acid. These observations suggest that the fate of browning participants such as chlorogenic acid during food processing should be taken into account in defining their role in the diet.

Potatoes also contain the steroidal glycosides α-chaconine and α-solanine. These sugars associated with the glycoalkaloids do not seem to participate in browning reactions since the glycoalkaloids were largely unaffected by processing.[44] However, we recently found a decrease of about 22% in tomatine content of green tomatoes after frying.[45] It is possible that this decrease may be due to browning reactions of the carbohydrate side chain of α-tomatine.

WHEAT PROTEINS

During baking, the mixture of water, protein and carbohydrates in dough is exposed to two distinct transformations. Desiccation of the surface on its exposure to temperatures reaching 215 °C results in the formation of a crust. The crust in turn encloses the bulk of dough in a steam phase at approximately 100 °C, forming the crumb. The nutritional impairment of gluten occurs particularly at the crust, which comprises nearly 50% of dry weight of whole bread. In hard biscuits, the bulk behaves thermally in a fashion similar to bread crust.[46-48]

In addition to its unique functional role in the formation of dough and the crumb and crust of bread and other foods, gluten is the major source of dietary protein in cereal products. The nutritional functionality of gluten may be impaired by its chemical reaction with other flour components including starch, the main component of flour.

Table 6.4. Effect of processing temperature on the nutritional value of cereal products. (Adapted from Ref. 49)

Product	Maximum processing temperature (°C)	PER	Nitrogen digestibility (%)
Puffed wheat	>260	−0.87	69
Wheat granules	204	0.36	80
Wheat flakes	149	0.46	72
Wheat shreds	121	1.67	75
Bread crust	175	0.62	85
Bread crumb	100	1.36	88
Wheat flour		1.11	89
Casein		3.27	94

Hansen *et al.*[49] studied the effects of thermal processing of wheat flour proteins on susceptibility to digestion and nutritional value. Table 6.4 shows that commercial wheat products such as puffed wheat which were heated at high temperatures had little protein nutritional value. In contrast, low-temperature processed products such as bread crumb and wheat shreds had minimal damage. They also found good correlations between lysine released by enzyme digestion and PER. The authors suggested that to maintain nutritive value, product temperature should not exceed 125 °C, as is the case for bread crumbs though not for bread crust.

Friedman and Finot[50] compared the growth of mice fed (a) an amino acid diet in which lysine was replaced by four dietary levels of γ-glutamyllysine; (b) wheat gluten diets fortified with lysine; (c) a wheat-bread-based diet (10% protein) supplemented before feeding with lysine or glutamyllysine, not co-baked; and (d) bread diets baked with these levels of lysine or γ-glutamyllysine. With the amino acid diet, the relative growth response to glutamyllysine was about half that of lysine. The effect of added lysine on the nutritional improvement of wheat gluten depended on both lysine and gluten concentrations in the diet. With 10 and 15% gluten, 0.37% lysine hydrochloride produced markedly increased weight gain.

The nutritive value of bread crust, fortified or not, was markedly less than that of crumb or whole bread. Lysine or γ-glutamyllysine at the highest level of fortification, 0.3%, improved the protein quality (PER) of crumb over that of either crust or whole bread, indicating a possible greater availability of the second limiting amino acid, threonine, in crumb. These data and additional metabolic studies with [U-^{14}C]γ-glutamyllysine suggest that γ-glutamyllysine, co-baked or not, is hydrolyzed in the kidneys and utilized *in vivo* as a source of lysine; it and related peptides merit further study as sources of lysine in low-lysine foods.

Our results also indicated that mice provide a good animal model to study protein quality of native, fortified and processed wheat proteins. In regard to labeling foods for protein nutritional quality, mouse bioassays have a major advantage. They require only about one-fifth of the test material needed for rat evaluations and can be completed in 14 days.

The following aspects of amino acid nutrition should be taken into account in assessing the nutritional value of glycated proteins. Amino acids are used both anabolically, as building blocks for protein biosynthesis, and catabolically, as energy sources. Catabolism for most amino acids proceeds through aminotransferase pathways; two exceptions are lysine and threonine. These nutritionally limiting amino acids are catabolized by nonaminitransferase-specific enzymes: threonine dehydratase acts on threonine and lysine ketoglutarate reductase on lysine. The concentrations of these enyzmes are subject to adaptive responses that control the utilization of these two amino acids.[50] Although both enzymes are induced by feeding diets high in protein, rats differ in the mechanism of the adaptive response to high-protein diets and to diets whose threonine or lysine content is less than that needed for growth. Thus reductase falls to very low levels in the liver of rats fed wheat gluten. This appears to be an adaptive response for conserving body lysine. At the same time, catabolism of body proteins increases, producing endogenous lysine needed for survival. These considerations imply that, as the level of wheat gluten or glycated, low-lysine protein in the diet decreases, lysine is no longer the limiting amino acid. Total protein or some other amino acid then becomes limiting.

NUTRITION OF MAILLARD PRODUCTS

For nutritional utilization, lysine must be liberated from a food protein by digestion. It is therefore important to establish factors that affect digestibility as well as the nutritional availability and safety of lysine derivatives formed in the Maillard and related reactions.[51-58]

Friedman and colleagues[14,59,60] studied the biological utilization of lysine derivatives in mice using all-amino acid diets in which all lysine was replaced by an equimolar amount of the derivative. Lysine derivatives were utilized to some extent as a nutritional source of lysine. The authors suggest that all such studies should use amino acid diets in which the derivatives can serve as the *only* source of lysine. This is not the case with glycated proteins.

Finot and colleagues[61-63] showed that the early Maillard product, deoxyketosyllysine (ε-N-fructosyllysine) was utilized by the rat as a source of lysine to the extent of about 5–15% compared to lysine. Hurrell and Carpenter[7] showed that protein-bound fructosyllysine formed in stored albumin–glucose mixtures did not serve as a lysine source.

Edersdobler and colleagues[64,65] studied dose–response excretion in humans of protein-bound ε-fructosyllysine. Glycated casein containing 0.8–5 g ε-fructosyllysine was consumed orally by 42 human volunteers. More than 90% of the lysine derivative was not recovered in the urine or feces. It may have been metabolized by microflora of the lower gastrointestinal tract, making it unavailable as a nutritional source of lysine.

Sherr *et al.*[66] showed that monofructosyllysine was absorbed in significant amounts by rats and incorporated into liver microsomes. In contrast, the difructosyllysine derivative was not absorbed to any extent. About 72% of absorbed monofructosyllysine competitively retarded the absorption of free lysine while the difructosyl derivative reduced lysine absorption by blocking the absorption site.

Plakas *et al.*[67] investigated the bioavailability of lysine in browned fish-protein isolate by measuring the lysine content in plasma of rainbow trout fed the isolate. They demonstrated an 80% loss in bioavailable lysine following heating the fish isolate under mild conditions (40 days at 37 °C). The authors concluded that rainbow trout are similar to other animals in their inability to utilize the deoxyketosyl (Amadori compound) of lysine formed in the early stages of the Maillard reaction and that the plasma response in trout was a good indicator of biologically available lysine.

These and related studies on structure-nutritional utilization of lysine derivatives suggest that not only steric bulk of the molecules but charge and basicity must influence the lysine derivatives' susceptibility to enzymatic hydrolysis and their transport and utilization as a nutritional source of lysine. With the advent of improved methods for isolation and characterization of such compounds, future studies should be directed toward a better assessment of their nutritional and toxicological significance.

PHYSIOLOGICAL EFFECTS OF MAILLARD PRODUCTS

Finot[61] offers a useful summary of physiological and pharmacological effects of Maillard products that may adversely affect protein, mineral and vitamin nutrition. Briefly, these symptoms include (a) inhibition of processes such as growth, protein and carbohydrate digestion, amino acid absorption and activity of intestinal enzymes including aminopeptidases, proteases and saccharidases, and pancreatic enzymes such as chymotrypsin; (b) induction of cellular changes in the kidneys (karyomegaly and hypertrophy), the liver (brown spots, hypertrophy and decrease in enzyme production) and the stomach cecum (hypertrophy); (c) adverse effects on mineral metabolism (Ca, Mg, Cu, Zn); and (d) variable effects on allergic response and cholesterol metabolism.

Von Wagenheim *et al.*[68] examined kidney histopathology of rats fed casein heated with glucose for 4 days at 65 °C. Enlarged epithelial cells and nuclei were observed after two weeks of feeding. The average size of the nuclei increased with feeding time, with significant differences being observed after 6, 8 or 10 weeks of feeding. The authors stated that the observed kidney damage is similar to that reported for lysinoalanine. The etiology of the effect is presently unknown, but would appear to be due to early or advanced stage browning products.[69]

Finot and Furniss[62] confirmed and extended the above findings about browning product-induced nephrotoxicity. They report that feeding either lysinoalanine or casein heated with glucose at 37 °C for 3 or 15 days induced nephrocytomegaly and was associated with urinary loss of Zn. Increased urinary loss of Cu was also reported. Kidney levels of Zn and Cu were higher than controls in the group fed heated casein–glucose. These observations suggest that alteration of the mineral content of the diet could minimize browning-induced kidney damage.[70–72]

In a related study,[16] we showed that the presence of glucose during alkaline treatment of soybean proteins significantly lessened the amount of lysinoalanine formed. A possible explanation for this effect is that glucose-blocked ε-NH_2 groups of lysine were unable to combine with dehydroalanine to form lysinoalanine. The potential of carbohydrates to prevent formation of kidney-damaging lysinoalanine merits further study.

The extent of severity of these effects will be influenced by the severity of the heat treatments, by the content and structure of different Maillard and crosslinked products formed on heating, and by the health and susceptibility of the consumer. We are challenged to define processing conditions to minimize the formation of the most antinutritional and toxic compounds. This will only be accomplished by detailed chemical and nutritional studies with specific, well-defined Maillard products that will permit defining a relative potency scale of antinutritional properties. It should then be possible to reduce the content of the most antinutritional ones in the diet.

PARENTERAL NUTRITION

Solutions used for intravenous nutrition, containing glucose–amino acid mixtures and glucose–protein hydrolysates, are often exposed to heat sterilization.[73] Stegink et al.[74] measured blood and urine levels of resulting Maillard reaction products in normal adult subjects nourished with sterilized parenteral solutions containing glucose and amino acids. Chromatograms showed a large number of ninhydrin-positive compounds in urine from these subjects. Oral consumption of the same solution, in contrast, did not result in these compounds. They also found that urinary Zn, Cu and Fe excretion increased two to five times above normal levels during intravenous infusion of the Maillard reaction products.

The authors concluded that fructosyl–amino acids produced by heat sterilization are either not absorbed during enteral feeding or are degraded in the intestinal mucosa before they can be absorbed. Possible adverse effects of liquid diets differ, depending on whether they are consumed by injection or orally. Parenteral consumption could lead to chelation of essential trace elements, resulting in adverse effects on mineral nutrition.[62]

ASCORBATE BROWNING

Sodium ascorbate (but not ascorbic acid) heated with wheat gluten and other proteins under conditions of crust baking, strongly inhibits the growth of mice when added to an otherwise nutritionally adequate diet.[48,75–80] Sodium ascorbate is widely used in many food applications. For example, the vitamin is added to flour before baking to improve bread-dough characteristics and to bacon to prevent nitrosamine formation.

In a related study Oste and Friedman[81] placed mice on a 14-day diet of nutritionally adequate casein supplemented at the expense of starch–dextrose with a 5% series of amino acids previously heated in the dry state with sodium ascorbate. Growth inhibition by the heated mixtures ranged from none for arginine to significant for tryptophan.

Elucidation of the nature and potency of the antinutritional material is needed (a) to reveal the extent to which concern for food safety is warranted and (b) to develop food processing conditions to prevent formation of toxic material.

BROWNING PREVENTION

Sulfur-containing amino acids such as cysteine, N-acetylcysteine and the tripeptide glutathione play key roles in the biotransformation of toxic compounds by actively participating in their detoxification. These antioxidant and antitoxic effects are due to a multiplicity of mechanisms including their ability to act as (a) reducing agents; (b) scavengers of reactive oxygen (free-radical species); (c) destroyers of fatty acid hydroperoxides; (d) strong nucleophiles which can trap electrophilic compounds and intermediates; (e) precursors for intracellular reduced glutathione; and (f) inducers of cellular detoxification.[82]

Thus, positive results were expected from an evaluation of the effectiveness of sulfur amino acids and sulfur-rich proteins (a) to prevent the formation of toxic browning products by trapping intermediates and (b) to reduce the toxicity of browning products in animals by preventing activation of such compounds to biologically active forms. These expectations were fulfilled, as evidenced by the following studies on the prevention of both enzymatic and nonenzymatic browning by sulfur amino acids.

β-Alanine, *N*-α-acetyl-L-lysine, glycyl–glycine and a mixture of amino acids were each heated with glucose in the absence and presence of the following potential inhibitors: *N*-acetyl-L-cysteine, L-cysteine, reduced glutathione, sodium bisulfite and urea. Inhibition of browning was measured as a function of temperature, time of heating and concentration of reactants. The results show that the SH compounds did indeed inhibit the Maillard reaction.[83–86] It should be possible to devise conditions to inhibit browning in amino acid–carbohydrate solutions used for parenteral nutrition.

Reflectance measurements were used to compare the relative effectiveness of a series of compounds in inhibition browning in freshly prepared and commercial fruit juices including apple, grape, grapefruit, orange and pineapple juices. For comparison, related studies were carried out with several protein-containing foods such as casein, barley flour, soy flour, nonfat dry milk and a commercial infant formula.[87–89]

Under certain conditions, SH-containing compounds may be as effective as sodium sulfite in preventing both enzymatic and nonenzymatic browning. Studies on the effects of concentration of inhibitors, storage conditions and pH revealed that *N*-acetyl-L-cysteine, cysteine ethyl and methyl esters, and reduced glutathione were nearly as effective on a molar basis as sodium sulfite in preventing browning of both apples and potatoes.[90] Would sulfur-rich proteins such as Bowman–Birk protease inhibitors from soybeans and purothionin from wheat[91] prevent Maillard reactions by trapping free radical intermediates?

In addition, Watanabe *et al.*[92] discovered that an extract from soil microorganisms catalyzed the deglycation of α- and ε-fructosyllysines to lysine. This finding suggests that these purified enzymes could be used to prevent or reverse Maillard reactions in foods and *in vivo*, provided they are safe in other regards. Practical applications of catechin browning inhibitors from tea extracts also merit study.[93]

In conclusion, future studies should define the prevention of browning and the consequent antinutritional and toxicological manifestations of browning products in whole foods as consumed. Whole foods include bread and other baked products, cereals, milk powders and other dairy products, fruits and fruit juices, salads, potatoes, meat, infant formulae and liquid diets. Such studies are especially important because the use of the widely used antibrowning compound, sodium sulfite, is being discontinued because many individuals are sensitive to it. Since Maillard and related reactions pervade many foods, potential benefits of preventing adverse consequences and optimizing beneficial ones of food browning to food quality and human health are significant.

ACKNOWLEDGEMENTS

The author thanks Linn U. Hansen, Talwinder S. Kahlon and Sigmund Schwimmer for reviewing this paper and his colleagues, whose names appear on the cited references, for excellent scientific collaboration.

REFERENCES

1. J. F. Cavins and M. Friedman, Automatic integration and computation of amino acid analyses, *Cereal Chem.*, **45**, 172–6 (1968).
2. G. Sarwar, R. Blair, M. Friedman, M. R. Gumbmann, L. R. Hackler and T. K. Smith, Comparison of interlaboratory variation in amino acid analysis and rat growth assays for evaluation of protein quality, *J. Assoc. Off. Anal. Chem.*, **68**, 52–6 (1985).
3. M. Friedman, Chemically reactive and unreactive lysine as an index of browning, *Diabetes*, **31** (Suppl. 3), 5–14 (1982).
4. K. J. Carpenter, Individual amino acid levels and bioavailability, in *Protein Quality in Humans: Assessment and In Vitro Estimation* (eds. C. E. Bodwell, J. S. Adkins and D. T. Hopkins), AVI, Westport, Connecticut, 1981, pp. 239–60.
5. J. W. Finley and M. Friedman, Chemical methods for available lysine, *Cereal Chem.*, **50**, 101–5 (1973).
6. M. Friedman, Effect of lysine modification on chemical, physical, nutritive, and functional properties of proteins, in *Food Proteins* (eds. J. R. Whitaker and S. R. Tannenbaum), AVI, Westport, Connecticut, 1977, pp. 446–83.
7. R. A. Hurrell and K. J. Carpenter, The reactive lysine content of heat-damaged material as measured in different ways, *Br. J. Nutr.*, **32**, 589–93 (1974).
8. M. Friedman and L. D. Williams, Stoichiometry of formation of Ruhemann's purple in the ninhydrin reaction, *Bioorg. Chem.*, **3**, 267–80 (1974).
9. M. Friedman, J. Pang and G. A. Smith, Ninhydrin-reactive lysine in food proteins, *J. Food Sci.*, **49**, 10–13, 20 (1984).
10. K. N. Pearce, D. Karahalios and M. Friedman, Ninhydrin assay for proteolysis in ripening cheese, *J. Food Sci.*, **52**, 432–5, 438 (1988).
11. R. E. Oste, Digestibility of processed food protein, in *Nutritional and Toxicological Consequences of Food Processing* (ed. M. Friedman), Plenum, New York, 1991, pp. 371–88.
12. S. S. Percival and B. O. Schneeman, Long term pancreatic response to feeding heat damaged casein in rats, *J. Nutr.*, **109**, 1609–14 (1971).
13. M. Friedman, J. C. Zahnley and P. M. Masters, Relationship between *in vitro* digestibility of casein and its content of lysinoalanine and D-amino acids, *J. Food Sci.*, **46**, 127–31 (1981).
14. M. Friedman, M. R. Gumbmann and L. Savoie, The nutritional value of lysinoalanine as a source of lysine, *Nutr. Repts. Int.*, **26**, 937–43 (1982).
15. M. Friedman, M. R. Gumbmann and P. M. Masters, Protein–alkali reactions: chemistry, toxicology, and nutritional consequences, *Adv. Exp. Med. Biol.*, **199**, 367–412 (1984).
16. M. Friedman, C. E. Levin and A. T. Noma, Factors governing lysinoalanine formation in soy proteins, *J. Food Sci.*, **49**, 1282–8 (1984).
17. M. Friedman, O. K. Grosjean and J. C. Zahnley, Carboxypeptidase inhibition of alkali-treated food proteins, *J. Agric. Food Chem.*, **33**, 208–13 (1985).

18. M. Friedman, O. K. Grosjean and J. C. Zahnley, Inactivation of metalloenzymes by food constituents, *Food Chem. Toxicol.*, **24**, 897–902 (1986).

19. J. C. Woodard, D. D. Short, M. R. Alvarez and J. Reyniers, Biologic effects of lysinoalanine, in *Protein Nutritional Quality of Foods and Feeds* (ed. M. Friedman), Part B, Marcel Dekker, New York, 1975, pp. 595–16.

20. M. Friedman, Glossary of nutritional terms, *Adv. Exp. Med. Biol.*, **105**, 841–63 (1978).

21. M. Friedman, Nutritional value of proteins from different food sources. A Review, *J. Agric. Food Chem.*, **44**, 1–24 (1996).

22. M. R. Gumbmann, M. Friedman and G. A. Smith, The nutritional values and digestibilities of heat-damaged casein and casein-carbohydrate mixtures, *Nutr. Repts. Int.*, **28**, 355–61 (1983).

23. G. A. Smith and M. Friedman, Effect of carbohydrates and heat on the amino acid composition and chemically available lysine content of casein, *J. Food Sci.*, **49**, 817–21 (1984).

24. N. V. Chuyen, N. Utsunomiya and H. Kato, Nutritional and physiological effects of casein modified by glucose under various conditions on growing adult rats, *Agric. Biol. Chem.*, **55**, 659–64 (1991).

25. B. Mori and H. Nakatsuji, Utilization in rats of ^{14}C-L-lysine-labeled casein browned by the amino-carbonyl reactions, *Agric. Biol. Chem.*, **41**, 345–50 (1977).

26. F. Evangelisti, C. Calcagno and P. Zuni, Relationship between blocked lysine and carbohydrate composition of infant formulas, *J. Food Sci.*, **59**, 335–7 (1994).

27. E. Lipka and Z. Ganowiak, Nutritional value of protein subjected to technological processing. Changes in content of the biologically active amino acids methionine, cysteine and taurine caused by sterilization, *Roczniki Panstwowego Zukladu Higieny*, **44**, 151–81 (1993); *Food Science and Technology Abstracts (FSTA)*, 7A97 (1994).

28. S. C. Keyes, P. Vincent and J. Hegarty, Effect of differential heat treatments on the protein quality of casein and lactalbumin, *J. Agric. Food Chem.*, **27**, 1405–7 (1979).

29. M. Tanaka, M. Kimiagar, T. C. Lee and C. O. Chichester, Effect of the Maillard reaction on the nutritional quality of protein, in *Protein Crosslinking: Nutritional and Medical Consequences* (ed. M. Friedman), Plenum, New York, 1977, pp. 321–41.

30. T. C. Lee, S. J. Pintauro and C. O. Chichester, Nutritional and toxicological effects of nonenzymatic Maillard browning, *Diabetes*, **31** (Suppl. 3), 37–46 (1982).

31. G. M. Dugan, M. R. Gumbmann and M. Friedman, Toxicological evaluation of Jimson weed (*Datura stramonium*) seed, *Food Chem. Toxicol.*, **27**, 501–10 (1989).

32. Y. Kato, T. Matsuda, N. Kato and R. Nakamura, Browning and protein polymerization induced by amino-carbonyl reaction of ovalbumin with glucose and lactose, *J. Agric. Food Chem.*, **36**, 806–9 (1984).

33. Y. Kato,, T. Matsuda, N. Kato, K. Watanabe and R. Nakamura, Browning and insolubilization of ovalbumin by the Maillard reaction with some aldohexoses, *J. Agric. Food Chem.*, **34**, 351–5 (1986).

34. J. E. Knipfel, H. G. Botting and J. M. McLaughlin, Nutritional quality of several proteins as affected by heating in the presence of carbohydrates, in *Protein Nutritional Quality of Foods and Feeds* (ed. M. Friedman), Part A, Marcel Dekker, New York, 1975, pp. 375–90.

35. K. S. Rhee and K. C. Rhee, Nutritional evaluation of the protein in oilseed products heated with sugars, *J. Food Sci.*, **46**, 164–8 (1981).

36. M. Friedman, Brandon, D. L., A. H. Bates and T. Hymowitz, Comparison of a commercial soybean cultivar and an isoline lacking the Kunitz trypsin inhibitor:

composition, nutritional value, and effect of heating, *J. Agric. Food Chem.*, **39**, 327–35 (1991).

37. M. Friedman, Composition and safety evaluation of potato berries, potato and tomato seeds, potatoes, and potato alkaloids, *ACS Symp. Ser.*, **484**, 429–62 (1992).

38. J. Sowokinos, Stress-induced transformation in carbohydrate metabolism, in *The Molecular and Cellular Biology of the Potato* (eds. M. J. Vayda and W. D. Park), CAB International, Wallingford, UK, 1990, pp. 137–58.

39. G. Marquez and M. C. Anon, Influence of reducing sugars and amino acids in the color development of fried potatoes, *J. Food Sci.*, **51**, 157–60.

40. S. Schwimmer, *Source Book of Food Enzymology*, AVI, Westport, Connecticut, 1981, pp. 119, 327.

41. L. Dao and M. Friedman, Chlorogenic acid content of fresh and processed potatoes determined by ultraviolet spectrophotometry, *J. Agric. Food Chem.*, **40**, 2152–6 (1992).

42. L. Dao and M. Friedman, Chlorophyll, chlorogenic acid, glycoalkaloids, and protease inhibitor content of fresh and green potatoes, *J. Agric. Food Chem.*, **42**, 633–9 (1994).

43. M. Friedman and L. Dao, Effect of autoclaving and conventional and microwave baking on the ergot alkaloid and chlorogenic acid content of morning glory (*Ipomoea tricolor Cav. cv.*) Heavenly Blue seeds, *J. Agric. Food Chem.*, **38**, 805–8 (1990).

44. M. Friedman and L. Dao, Distribution of glycoalkaloids in potato plants and commercial potato products, *J. Agric. Food Chem.*, **40**, 419–23 (1992).

45. M. Friedman and C. E. Levin, α-Tomatine content of tomato and tomato products determined by HPLC with pulsed amperometric detection, *J. Agric. Food Chem.*, **43**, 1507–11 (1995).

46. A. A. Betschart, Improving protein quality of bread — nutritional benefits and realities, in *Improvement in the Nutritional Quality of Foods and Feeds* (ed. M. Friedman), Plenum, New York, 1978, pp. 703–34.

47. M. Friedman, Dietary impact of food processing, *Ann. Rev. Nutr.*, **12**, 119–37 (1992).

48. I. I. Ziderman and M. Friedman, Thermal and compositional changes of dry wheat gluten–carbohydrate mixtures during simulated crust baking, *J. Agric. Food Chem.*, **33**, 1096–102 (1985).

49. L. P. Hansen, P. H. Johnston and R. E. Ferrel, The assessment of thermal processing of wheat flour proteins by physical, chemical, and enzymatic methods, in *Protein Nutritional Quality of Foods and Feeds* (ed. M. Friedman), Part B, Marcel Dekker, New York, pp. 393–415.

50. M. Friedman and P. A. Finot, Nutritional improvement of bread with lysine and glutamyl-lysine, *J. Agric. Food Chem.*, **38**, 2011–20 (1990).

51. J. E. Ford and C. Shorrock, Metabolism of heat-damaged proteins in the rat, *Br. J. Nutr.*, **26**, 311–22 (1971).

52. M. Fujimaki, S. Homma, N. Arakawa and C. Inagaki, Growth response of rats fed with a diet containing nondialyzable melanoidin, *Agric. Biol. Chem.*, **43**, 497–503 (1979).

53. R. F. Hurrell, Influence of the Maillard reaction on the nutritional value of foods, in *The Maillard Reaction in Food Processing, Human Nutrition, and Physiology* (ed. P. A. Finot, H. U. Aeschbacher, R. F. Hurrell and P. Liardon), Birkhauser, Basel, Switzerland, 1990, pp. 245–58.

54. R. F. Hurrell and P. A. Finot, Nutritional consequences of the reactions between proteins and oxidized polyphenols, in *Nutritional and Toxicological Aspects of Food Safety* (ed. M. Friedman), Plenum, New York, pp. 423–35.

55. J. Mauron, Influence of processing on nutritional quality, *J. Nutr. Sci. Vitaminol.*, **36**, S57–S69 (1990).

56. A. Poiffait and J. Adrian, Interaction between casein and vitamin A during food processing, in *Nutritional and Toxicological Consequences of Food Processing* (ed. M. Friedman), Plenum, New York, 1991, pp. 61–73.

57. E. Quattrucci, Heat treatments and nutritional significance of Maillard reaction products, in *Nutritional and Toxicological Aspects of Food Safety* (eds. R. Walker and E. Quattrucci), Taylor & Francis, London, 1988, pp. 113–23.

58. S. A. Varnish and K. J. Carpenter, Mechanisms of heat damage in proteins. 6. The digestibility of individual amino acids in heated and propionylated proteins, *Br. J. Nutr.*, **34**, 339–49 (1975).

59. M. Friedman and M. R. Gumbmann, Biological availability of ε-N-methyl-L-lysine, 1-N-methyl-L-histidine, and 3-N-methyl-L-histidine in mice, *Nutr. Repts Int.*, **19**, 437–43 (1979).

60. M. Friedman and M. R. Gumbmann, Bioavailability of some lysine derivatives in mice, *J. Nutr.*, **111**, 1362–9 (1981).

61. P. A. Finot, Metabolism and physiological effects of Maillard reaction products, in *The Maillard Reaction in Food Processing, Human Nutrition, and Physiology* (eds. P. A. Finot, H. U. Aeschbacher, R. F. Hurrell and R. Liardon), Birkhauser, Basel, Switzerland, 1990, pp. 259–71.

62. P. A. Finot and E. E. Furniss, Nephrocytomegaly in rats induced by Maillard reaction products: the involvement of metal ions, in *Amino-Carbonyl Reactions in Food and Biological Systems* (ed. M. Fujimaki), Elsevier, Amsterdam, The Netherlands, 1986, pp. 493–502.

63. P. A. Finot, E. Bujard, F. Mottu and J. Mauron, Availability of the true Schiff's base of lysine and lactose in milk, in *Protein Crosslinking: Nutritional and Medical Consequences* (ed. M. Friedman), Plenum, New York, 1977, pp. 343–64.

64. H. F. Ebersdobler, A. Gross, U. Klusman and K. Schlecht, Absorption and metabolism of heated protein–carbohydrate mixtures in humans, in *Absorption and Utilization of Amino Acids* (ed. M. Friedman), Boca Raton, Florida, Vol. 3, 1989, pp. 91–102.

65. H. F. Ebersdobler, M. Lohmann and K. Buhl, Utilization of early Maillard reaction products in humans, in *Nutritional and Toxicological Consequences of Food Processing* (ed. M. Friedman), Plenum, New York, 1991, pp. 363–70.

66. B. Sherr, C. M. Lee and C. Jelesciewicz, Absorption and metabolism of lysine Maillard products in relation to utilization of L-lysine, *J. Agric. Food Chem.*, **37**, 119–22 (1989).

67. S. Plakas, T. C. Lee and R. E. Wolke, Bioavailability of lysine in Maillard browned protein as determined by plasma lysine response in rainbow trout (*Salmo gairdneri*), *J. Nutr.*, **118**, 19–22 (1988).

68. B. Von Wagenheim, T. Hanichen and H. H. Ebersdobler, Histopathological investigation of the rat kidneys after feeding heat damaged proteins, *Z. Enahrungswiss.*, **23**, 219–29 (1984).

69. J. O'Brien and R. Walker, Toxicological effects of dietary Maillard reaction products in the rat, *Food Chem. Toxicol.*, **26**, 775–84 (1988).

70. M. Friedman and K. N. Pearce, Copper (II) and cobalt (II) affinities of LL- and LD-lysinoalanine diasteromers: implications for food safety and nutrition, *J. Agric. Food Chem.*, **37**, 123–7 (1989).

71. K. N. Pearce and M. Friedman, The binding of copper (II) and other metal ions by lysinoalanine and related compounds and its significance for food safety, *J. Agric. Food Chem.*, **36**, 707–817 (1988).
72. G. Rehner and Th. Walter, Effect of Maillard products and lysinoalanine on the bioavailability of iron, copper, and zinc, *Z. Ernahrungswiss.*, **30**, 50–5 (1991).
73. T. P. Labuza and S. A. Massaro, Browning and amino acid loss in model total parenteral nutrition solutions, *J. Food Sci.*, **55**, 821–6 (1990).
74. L. D. Stegink, J. B. Freeman, L. Den Besten and J. Filer, Maillard reaction products in parenteral nutrition, *Prog. Food Nutr. Sci.*, **5**, 265–78 (1981).
75. J. Dunn, M. U. Ahmet, M. H. Murtishaw, J. M. Richardson, M. D. Walla, S. R. Thrope and J. W. Baynes, Reaction of ascorbate with lysine and protein under autooxidizing conditions: formation of *N*-ε-(carboxymethyl)lysine by reaction between lysine and products of autooxidation of ascorbate, *Biochem.*, **29**, 10964–70 (1990).
76. M. Friedman, M. R. Gumbmann and I. I. Ziderman, Nutritional value and safety in mice of proteins and their admixtures with carbohydrates and vitamin C after heating, *J. Nutr.*, **117**, 508–18 (1987).
77. M. Friedman, M. R. Gumbmann and I. I. Ziderman, Nutritional and toxicological consequences of browning during simulated crust-baking, in *Protein Quality and Effects of Processing* (eds. R. D. Phillips and J. W. Finley), Marcel Dekker, New York, 1989, pp. 189–217.
78. M. Friedman, R. E. Wilson and I. I. Ziderman, Mutagen formation in heated wheat gluten, carbohydrates, and gluten/carbohydrate blends, *J. Agric. Food Chem.*, **38**, 1019–28 (1990).
79. R. E. Oste, D. L. Brandon, A. H. Bates and M. Friedman, Effect of the Maillard reaction of the Kunitz soybean trypsin inhibitor on its interaction with monoclonal antibodies, *J. Agric. Food Chem.*, **38**, 258–61 (1990).
80. I. I. Ziderman, K. S. Gregorski, S. V. Lopez and M. Friedman, Thermal interaction of vitamin C with proteins in relation to nonenzymatic browning of foods and Maillard reactions, *J. Agric. Food Chem.*, **37**, 1480–6 (1989).
81. R. E. Oste and M. Friedman, Safety of heated amino acid–sodium ascorbate blends, *J. Agric. Food Chem.*, **38**, 1687–90 (1990).
82. M. Friedman, Improvement in the safety of foods by SH-containing amino acids and peptides. A review, *J. Agric. Food Chem.*, **42**, 3–20 (1994).
83. M. Friedman, Prevention of adverse effects of food browning, *Adv. Exp. Med. Biol.*, **289**, 171–216 (1991).
84. M. Friedman and J. L. Cuq, Chemistry, analysis, nutritional value, and toxicology of tryptophan. A review, *J. Agric. Food Chem.*, **36**, 1079–93 (1988).
85. M. Friedman and I. Molnar-Perl, Inhibition of food browning by sulfur amino acids. Part 1. Heated amino acid–glucose systems, *J. Agric. Food Chem.*, **38**, 1642–7 (1990).
86. J. T. MacGregor, J. D. Tucker, I. I. Ziderman, C. M. Wehr, R. R. Wilson and M. Friedman, Nonclastogenicity in mouse bone marrow of fructose/lysine and other sugar/amino acid browning products with *in vitro* genotoxicity, *Food Chem. Toxicol.*, **27**, 715–21 (1989).
87. M. Friedman, I. Molnar-Perl and D. K. Knighton, Browning prevention in fresh and dehydrated potatoes by SH-containing amino acids, *Food Addit. Contam.*, **9**, 499–503 (1992).
88. I. Molnar-Perl and M. Friedman, Inhibition of food browning by sulfur amino acids. Part 2. Fruit juices and protein-containing foods, *J. Agric. Food Chem.*, **38**, 1648–51 (1990).

89. I. Molnar-Perl and M. Friedman, Inhibition of food browning by sulfur amino acids. Part 3. Apples and potatoes, *J. Agric. Food Chem.*, **38**, 1652–6 (1990).

90. M. Friedman and F. F. Bautista, Inactivation of polyphenol oxidase by thiols in the absence and presence of potato tissue suspensions, *J. Agric. Food Chem.*, **43**, 69–76 (1995).

91. D. L. Brandon, A. H. Bates and M. Friedman, Antigenicity of soybean protease inhibitors, in *Protease Inhibitors as Cancer Chemopreventive Agents* (eds. W. Troll and A. R. Kennedy), Plenum, New York, 1993, pp. 107–29.

92. N. Watanabe, M. Ohtsuka, S. I. Takahashi, Y. Sakano and D. Fukimoto, Enzymatic deglycation of fructosyl-lysine, *Agric. Biol. Chem.*, **51**, 1063–4 (1987).

93. N. Kinae, M. Yamashita, S. Esaki and S. Kamiya, Inhibitory effects of tea extracts on the formation of advanced glycosylated products, in *The Maillard Reaction in Food Processing, Human Nutrition, and Physiology* (eds. P. A. Finot, H. U. Aeschbacher, R. F. Hurrell and R. Liardon), Birkhauser, Basel, Switzerland, 1990, pp. 221–6.

7

Genotoxicity of Maillard Reaction Products

JON W. WONG and TAKAYUKI SHIBAMOTO

Department of Environmental Toxicology,
University of California Davis, California, USA

The chemical pathways between amines and reducing sugars lead to a complex mixture of products. The Maillard reaction, or nonenzymatic browning, is a set of reactions responsible for providing cooked foods with their color, flavor and aroma. In addition, Maillard reaction products have also been investigated for nutritional, physiological and biological activities. The processes and products of the Maillard reaction have been implicated in a wide variety of diseases such as diabetes and cancer, and pathological conditions such as aging. In this chapter, the formation and genotoxic testing of mutagenic Maillard reaction products in model and food systems will be reviewed.

TESTS FOR GENOTOXICITY

The mutagenic activity of foods and food components as well as other mutagens have been studied in a number of test systems using bacteria (*Salmonella typhimurium, Escherichia coli*), fungi (*Saccharomyces cerevisiae*), insects (*Drosophila melanogaster*) and mammalian species *in vitro* (Chinese hamster ovary cells) and *in vivo* (mouse). The three major test systems as categorized by Anderson (1988) for mutagenicity testing are gene mutations, chromosomal damage and DNA damage/repair. Gene mutations consist of substitutions, deletions or insertions of one or more nucleotide base pairs in DNA and are detected by characteristics controlled by specific gene loci (i.e. histidine independence, arabinose resistance, 8-azaguanine resistance, adenine

The Maillard Reaction: Consequences for the Chemical and Life Sciences. Edited by Raphael Ikan
©1996 John Wiley & Sons Ltd

biosynthesis, hypoxanthine guanine phosphoribosyl transferase activity). Chromosomal damage is detected by cytological and genetic methods to identify variations in the number (aneuploidy and polyploidy) and structure of the chromosomes. DNA damage/repair is the ability of the genome to repair itself (excision, post-replication, recombination repair) after it is damaged. Detection is measured by DNA repair in wild-type and DNA repair-deficient bacteria, unscheduled DNA synthesis, DNA breakage, mitotic recombination, gene conversion and sister chromatid exchange. All three tests systems have been used in evaluating Maillard reaction products, but the *Salmonella/* mutagenicity (Ames) assay has been the commonly used method to determine gene mutation.

In the *Salmonella*/mutagenicity (Ames) assay (Ames *et al.*, 1975; Maron and Ames, 1983), compounds are tested on petri dishes containing specially constructed histidine-requiring mutants of *Salmonella typhimurium* that are reverted to prototrophy by a mutagenic compound. The assay consists of a liver homogenate fraction (S9) mix, prepared from animals (usually rats) dosed with phenobarbital or Arochlor to increase the rate of enzymatic metabolism toward the agent. Bacterial tester strains have been developed for base-pair mutations (purine–purine, pyrimidine–pyrimidine base-pair transitions or purine–pyrimidine, pyrimidine–purine base-pair transversion) using the *S. typhimurium* strains TA153 and frameshift mutations (addition or deletion of a base in DNA) using the strains TA1537 and TA1538. Other more sensitive strains such as TA98 and TA100 are less specific to the type of mutation caused. Table 7.1 lists the mutagenic potential of some heterocyclic aromatic amines isolated from foods and formed from the Maillard reaction toward *S. typhimurium* strains TA98 and TA100 with S9 microsomal activation. Some of

Table 7.1. Mutagenic activity of heterocyclic aromatic amines found in foods in *Salmonella typhimurium* strains TA98 and TA100 with S9 microsomal activation. Refer to Tables 7.4 and 7.5 for identification of the mutagenic compound. (Adapted from Sugimura, 1986, Sugimura *et al.*, 1993 and Overvik *et al.*, 1993.)

	Number of revertants	
Mutagen	TA98	TA100
IQ	433000	7000
MeIQ	661000	30000
IQx	75000	1500
MeIQx	145000	14000
4,8-DiMeIQx	183000–206000	8000
7,8-DiMeIQx	163000–189000	9900
PhIP	1800–2000	120
Aflatoxin B_i	6000	28000
Benzo[a]pyrene	320	660

these food mutagens, such as IQ and MeIQ, exhibit strong mutagenic activity toward *S. typhimurium*, with S9 activation in comparison to well-known carcinogens such as aflatoxin B_1 and benzo[a]pyrene.

THE MAILLARD REACTION AND ITS MUTAGENIC PRODUCTS IN MODEL SYSTEMS

The initial, intermediate and final stages of the Maillard reaction are shown in Figure 7.1. The early stages of the Maillard reaction begin with the condensation of a primary amine from an amino acid or protein and a carbonyl such as glucose, fructose, maltose, lactose or some reducing sugar. The intermediate stages involving the degradation of the Amadori compound and its subsequent mechanisms form a variety of intermediate products and precursors. The final stages of the Maillard reaction are complex and involve the condensation of many low molecular weight intermediates and products into high molecular weight polymers or melanoidins. Although the melanoidins are the final products of the browning reaction, many low molecular species such as amines, carbonyls, furfurals, fission products and reductones are formed. Many of these products are very important in their sensory and biological activities. Of these products, O'Brien and Morrissey (1989) have classified these mainly volatile compounds into three groups:

- Simple sugar dehydration/fragmentation products (furans, pyrones, cyclopentenes, carbonyls, acids)
- Simple amino acid degradation products (aldehydes and sulfur compounds)
- Compounds produced by further reactions (pyrroles, pyridines, imidazoles, pyrazines, oxazoles, thiazoles, aldol condensation products)

Hodge (1953) indicated that simple model systems could be used to study nonenzymatic browning reactions that are found in complex food systems. Model systems of simple amine and carbonyl systems have been used to study the nature of cooked foods such as pigment characterization, isolation and identification of volatiles, antioxidative activity, sensory profiles and mutagenic activity (Shibamoto, 1982). Studies of the mutagenic activity of sugar/amino acid heated systems provide useful models in the elucidation of the mutagenic Maillard reaction products found in heated food systems. Typical model systems used for various mutagenic studies are shown in Table 7.2. The components of the model browning systems can be determined if they are mutagenic, antimutagenic or neutral in genotoxicity tests such as the *Salmonella*/Ames assay.

Spingarn and Garvie (1979) investigated the browning reaction of sugars (arabinose, 2-deoxyglucose, galactose, glucose, rhamnose and xylose) and

132

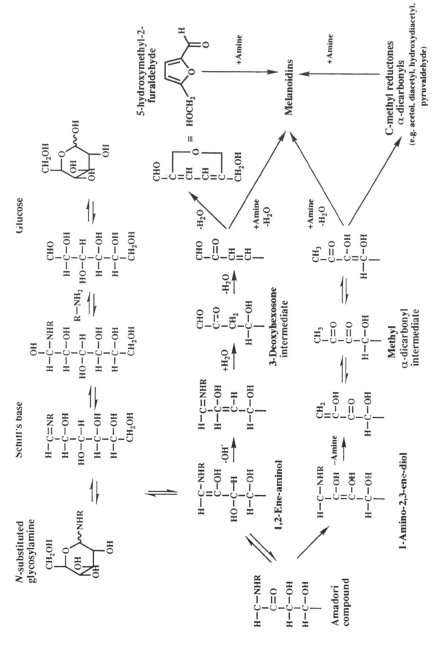

Figure 7.1 The Maillard reaction and degradation pathway of Amadori compounds. (Adapted from O'Brien and Morrissey, 1989, and Powrie *et al.*, 1986)

Table 7.2. Maillard reaction model systems used to study mutagenicity

System	Reference	Summary of research
Sugar/ammonia	Spingarn and Garvie (1979)	Reaction of sugars with ammonium ion under reflux conditions results in strong mutagenic activity, pyrazine derivatives formed
Glucose/cysteamine	Mihara and Shibamoto (1980)	Isolation of thiazolidines showed mutagenic activity toward *S. typhimurium* strains TA98 and TA100 with and without S9 mix
Cyclotene/ammonia	Shibamoto and Bernhard (1980)	Polycyclic pyrazines identified from browning systems, compounds shown to have mutagenic activity
Glucose/lysine	Shinohara *et al.* (1980)	Mutagenicity of browning mixture on *S. typhimurium* TA100
Glucose/albumin	Pintauro *et al.* (1980)	Ames mutagenicity tests found no mutagenic activity in lipid- and water-soluble fractions of a protein/sugar browning solution
Sugar/ammonia	Stich *et al.* (1981a, 1981b)	Mutagenic activity observed subjected CHO cells, *S. cerevisiae* strain D7, and *Salmonella* strains TA98 and TA100 with and without S9 mix and detected mutagenic activity
Glucose/amino acids Fructose/amino acids	Powrie *et al.* (1981)	Assessed three short-term tests to assess the clastogenic and point mutagenic activities of browning solutions; pH dependence in mutagenic activity, observed chromosomal aberrations in CHO cells, mitotic recombination and mutation in *S. cerevisiae* strain D5; induction of histidine prototrophy occurrence in *Salmonella* strains GA98 and TA100 without S9 mix
Rhamnose/ ammonia/H_2S	Toda *et al.* (1981)	Dichloromethane extract of browning solution exhibited strong mutagenicity, further fractionation of the extract showed the presence of alkylimidazoles
Maltol/ammonia	Shibamoto *et al.* (1981)	Mutagenicity isolated in various fractions, components in fractions isolated by GC/MS

continued

Table 7.2. *Continued*

System	Reference	Summary of research
Starch/glycine	Wei *et al.* (1981)	Baking model system of starch and glycine exhibited dose-related mutagenicity, but heated starch system did not possess mutagenic activity
Fructose/lysine	Chan *et al.* (1982)	Antimutagenic effects of heated fructose/lysine solution and caramelized sucrose toward the aflatoxin and nitrosamines
Various sugars/ various amino acids mixtures	Omura *et al.* (1983)	Mutagens identified in MRPs of 20 different amino acids with various sugars; several mutagens identified
Glucose/amino acid Amino acid pyrolysis Protein/starch	Spingarn *et al.* (1983)	Stoichiometry correlation and structural requirements for mutagenicity requirements; possible inhibitory effect of mutagen formation in starchy systems
Diacetyl/ammonia	Shibamoto (1983)	No mutagenic activity observed in major flavor compounds such as alkylimidazoles
Fructose/glycine, alanine/creatinine	Nyhammar *et al.* (1986)	IQ and MeIQx are major mutagens isolated from glycine system, while 4,8-DiMeIQx is the main mutagen isolated from the alanine system
Ribose/amino acids	Gazzani *et al.* (1987)	MRPs from ribose–lysine shows higher mutagenic activity than glucose–lysine systems
Creatine or creatinine/glycine/ sugars	Skog and Jagerstad (1990)	Effects of monosaccharides and dissacharides in the formation of heterocyclic aromatic amines; inhibition of mutagen formation by excess sugars and MRPs
Fructose/arginine Fructose/glycine Fructose/lysine Fructose/tryptophan Glucose/Arg, Gly, Lys or Trp Xylose/ Arg, Gly, Lys or Trp	Yen *et al.* (1992)	Antioxidative activity of xylose/amino acid browning mixtures; strong inhibition by mutagenicity of sugars/Trp and xylose/amino acids toward IQ, Trp-P-1 and Glu-P-1; enhanced mutagenicity by fructose/Gly and fructose/Arg toward Trp-P-1
Glucose/creatinine/ glucose/$FeSO_4$	Johansson and Jagerstad (1993)	Addition of iron doubled the formation of MeIQx in model meat system

continued

Table 7.2. *Continued*

System	Reference	Summary of research
Creatinine/glucose/ threonine	Skog and Jagerstad (1993)	Incorporation of [1-^{14}C] or [6-^{14}C]glucose into model systems demonstrates that glucose is an important precursor in mutagen formation in foods
Xylose/lysine Creatinine/glucose	Yen and Chau (1993) Yen and Hsieh (1994)	Inhibition of MeIQx by MRPs in a glycine model system; antimutagenic effects of MRPs toward IQ and IQ metabolites
Glucose/amino acid	Hiramoto *et al.* (1994)	DNA breaking activity observed with MRPs of glucose and amino acids (Ala, Arg, Cys, Gly, His, Lys, Pro)

ammonia refluxed 30–120 min at 100°C. The organic solvent extract from the browning solution was mutagenic on *S. typhimurium* strains TA98 and TA100 with S9 activation. They investigated the correlation between mutagenicity and pyrazine formation, though the pyrazines themselves were not mutagenic.

Powrie *et al.* (1981) used three tests to investigate the clastogenic and mutagenic activities of arginine, lysine, histidine, serine, glutamine and glutamic acid with either glucose or fructose. The Maillard reaction products produced in these systems increase chromosomal aberrations in Chinese hamster cells with S9 activation, mitotic recombination in *Saccharomyces cerevisiae* strain D5 and induction of histidine revertants in *S. typhimurium* strain TA100 without S9 activation.

Shibamoto *et al.* (1981) showed that the browning reaction products between maltol and ammonia were mutagenic in the tester strain TA98 with S9 activation. Maltol is formed from simple sugars or carbohydrates and is also shown to possess mutagenic activity (Bjeldanes and Chew, 1979). A fractionated extract from the reaction of maltol and ammonia formed from proteins or amino acids during heat treatment exhibited mutagenic activity and contained 2-ethyl-3-hydroxy-6-methylpyridine, acetamide, 2,3-dimethylpyrazine, unreacted maltol and unknown pyridine derivates as the major constituents. Although this fraction exhibited strong mutagenicity, authentic samples of the major components, 2-ethyl-3-hydroxy-6-methylpyridine and acetamide did not exhibit any mutagenic activity toward tester strains TA98 and TA100 with S9 activation.

Omura *et al.* (1983) studied the mutagens produced by Maillard reactions of equimolar amounts of 20 different amino acids with sugars refluxed for 10 h at

100°C. The mutagenic activity varied with the nature of amino acids, sugars and the presence and absence of S9 microsomal activation in the tester strains (*Salmonella typhimurium* TA100 and TA98). No mutagenic activity was detected with the browned solutions of glucose with tryptophan, dicysteine, tyrosine, aspartic acid, asparagine or glutamic acid. Mutagenic activity was observed on TA100 strain without S9 activation for most amino acids but decreased in the presence of S9 activation. Mutagenic activity was not observed with leucine, serine, threonine, methionine and glutamic acid, but activity was observed with arginine, glycine, alanine, valine and isoleucine on TA98 strain with S9 activation. Glucose and cysteine products showed mutagenicity on both strains and were enhanced by S9 activation. Other browning experiments showed that fructose, galactose and xylose formed mutagens with all amino acids with the exception of tryptophan. Other factors that determine mutagen formation were pH and heating time. A browning sample at pH 7 between glucose and phenylalanine showed the highest mutagenicity on TA100. Most of the mutagens were low molecular weight intermediates of the Maillard reaction between glucose and phenylalanine, lysine and cysteine.

Gazzani *et al.* (1987) studied the mutagenic activities of Maillard reaction products of several amino acids with ribose or glucose. High revertants in *S. typhimurium* TA98 and TA100 strains with and without S9 mix were observed. While the amino acids, arginine, glutamate and isoleucine showed little mutagenicity, other amino acids produced in the Maillard reaction with ribose such as alanine, asparagine, aspartate, cysteine, cystine, glycine, leucine, methionine, phenylalanine, proline, hydroxyproline, serine, threonine and valine were mutagenic in the TA100 strain. The mutagenic activity of ribose was generally higher than that in glucose, and lysine was shown to be the most active amino acid in the production of mutagenic compounds.

MUTAGENICITY OF ISOLATED MAILLARD REACTION PRODUCTS AND THEIR PRECURSORS

Since Maillard reaction products were not well known for many years, it was not until advanced developments in analytical instrumentation and identification techniques enabled investigators to isolate and identify individual components. In the 1960s, paper and thin layer chromatography methods were applied to isolate browning products, but due to the low resolution of these methods, the compounds isolated were limited to rather high boiling point compounds such as alkylhydroxyimidazoles (Shibamoto, 1983). Heterocyclic compounds such as imidazole and pyrrole derivatives were identified in Maillard reactions by the end of the 1960s. Despite the early research, the investigations of individual reaction products were stimulated by the development of gas chromatography, high-performance liquid chromatography and mass spectrometry during the 1970s and 1980s (Shibamoto, 1989). The use of GC/MS (gas chromatography/mass spectrometry) techniques, for instance, allowed for the identification of nearly one hundred volatile components from an L-rhamnose/ammonia browning model system (Shibamoto and Bernhard, 1978). Gas chromatography was beginning to be used to study browning reaction products in the 1970s when flavor development led to the discovery of many heterocyclic compounds such as furans, thiophenes, thiazoles, pyrazines, pyrroles, imidazoles and oxazoles. Since the 1980s, extensive mutagenicity testing on the products of Maillard browning model systems has been conducted.

DICARBONYL COMPOUNDS

Dicarbonyl compounds such as maltol and glyoxal are present in coffee, soybeans, baked cereals and bread crusts. Nagao *et al.* (1986) isolated glyoxal (**1**), methylglyoxal (**2**) and ethylglyoxal (**3**) in bourbon, brandy, wine, sake, coffee, tea, soft drinks, bread, toast, soy sauce and soybean paste. Of the liquids, soy sauce contained the largest amounts of glyoxal, methylglyoxal and ethylglyoxal at 4.9, 8.7 and 8.4 μg/mL, respectively, whereas tea (black and green) and soft drinks contained the least or only trace amounts. Bjeldanes and Chew (1979) investigated the 1,2-dicarbonyl compounds, diacetyl (**4**), maltol (**5**) and glyoxal, and found that they were mutagenic in *S. typhimurium* strains TA98 and TA100 with and without S9 activation. Similarly, Yamaguchi and Nakagawa (1983) determined that various trioses and glyoxal derivatives such as dihydroxyacetone (**6**), glyceraldehyde (**7**), glyoxal, methyl glyoxal and glyoxylic acid (**8**) were mutagenic in *S. typhimurium* strain TA100 without S9 activation.

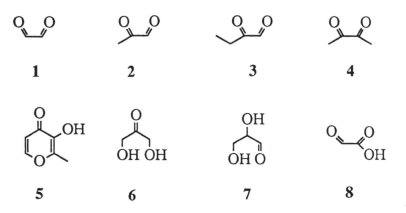

FURANS AND FURFURALS

Shinohara *et al.* (1986) demonstrated that furans are weakly mutagenic in the *Salmonella*/microsomal assay in comparison to other strong mutagens such as benzo[a]pyrene. 5-Hydroxymethyl-2-furaldehyde (**9**; 5-HMF), furfural (**10**), and 5-methylfurfural (**11**; 5-MF) were formed and identified from reactions of sugars with amino acids (lysine–arabinose, arginine–arabinose, lysine–xylose and arginine–xylose) at 100 °C for 4 h. These furan compounds were mutagenic in *S. typhimurium* strain TA100 with S9 activation and possessed DNA breaking activity in the presence of Cu^{2+}. 5-HMF was shown to possess the strongest mutagenicity, while the nonaldehyde-containing furans were shown to possess weaker activities. Similarly, Omura *et al.* (1983) observed mutagenicity from an ethanol extract of a browned solution of glucose and phenylalanine using the *Salmonella*/microsomal assay. 5-HMF was isolated in the extract by column chromatography and identified by ultraviolet and nuclear magnetic resonance spectroscopies and mass spectrometry. However, Kong *et al.* (1989) studied the effects of furans and furfurals on the mutagenic activity on the heterocyclic aromatic compounds 3-amino-1,4-dimethyl-5*H*-pyrido[4,3-*b*]indole (Trp-P-1) and benzo[a]pyrene (B[a]P) in *S. typhimurium* strains TA98 and TA100. The furan compounds, 5-HMF, 5-MF, furfural, furfuryl alcohol (**12**), furan (**13**), 2-acetylfuran (**14**) and 2-methylfuran (**15**) were shown to inhibit the mutagenicities of Trp-P-1, B[a]P and 2-aminoflur-orene toward *S. typhimurium* TA98 and TA100 strains in the presence of S9 activation. 5-HMF, furfural and 2-acetylfuran were more effective inhibitors, while furan and 2-methylfuran were the least. This work suggests an important role of carbonyls in the dual functionality of mutagenicity and desmutagenicity of furans as well as complexities of Maillard reaction product interactions in food systems.

PYRROLES

Pyrroles have been isolated in various food systems and some of them are important in the flavors of beverages, ice cream, candy and puddings (Maga *et al.*, 1981). Omura *et al.* (1983) isolated two compounds, 5-HMF and the pyrrole compound, ε-(2-formyl-5-hydroxymethyl)pyrrol-1-yl-(norleucine) (**16**), from a mutagenic fraction of a glucose and lysine browning mixture. Yen and Lee (1986) evaluated the mutagenic activities of three carbonyl-containing pyrroles commonly formed in Maillard reaction mixtures. In the Ames assay, 2-acetylpyrrole (**17**), pyrrole-2-carboxaldehyde (**18**) and pyrrole-2-carboxylic acid (**19**) were shown not to be mutagenic in the tester strains TA97, TA98, TA100, TA102 and TA104, with and without S9 activation. However, when these pyrroles were reacted with nitrite at acidic conditions (pH 3) at 50 °C for 24 h, the 2-acetylpyrrole–nitrite mixture showed strong mutagenicity in all tester strains. The other two pyrrole–nitrite mixtures possessed minimum or no mutagenic responses. The formation of the mutagenic products varied with pH, heating time, and nitrite and pyrrole concentrations. This work suggests that the presence of the carbonyl group in 2-acetylpyrrole influences the mutagenic strength of nitrosylated pyrrole compounds.

DITHIANES

Lee *et al.* (1994a, 1994b) identified the compounds 1,3-dithiane (**20**) and 1,4-dithiane (**21**) extracted from pork juice and studied the mutagenic activities in the *Salmonella* microsomal test and in the Chinese hamster ovary cell line. Other Maillard reaction products such as pyrazines, pyridines, furans, pyrroles, thiophenes, thiazoles and imidazoles were also tested and compared. 1,3-Dithiane exhibited the strongest mutagenic activity in *S. typhimurium* strains TA98 and TA100 with and without S9 activation, but 1,4-dithiane and other thiazoles were weakly mutagenic, with similar activity to that of 2,6-dimethylpyrazine. The sulfur compounds had similar mutagenic responses to other browning products such as hydroxymethylfurfural and methylglyoxal but have not been shown to be carcinogenic.

THIAZOLIDINES AND *N*-NITROSOTHIAZOLIDINES

Thiazolidines are important Maillard reaction products when sugars react with sulfur-containing amines, amino acids or proteins (Umano *et al.*, 1984). Mihara and Shibamoto (1980) isolated several fractions from a heated cysteamine–glucose browning system and tested the mutagenic activity in the tester strains TA98 and TA100 with and without S9 activation. In a methylene chloride extract, unsubstituted (22), 2-n-methyl- (23), 2-n-ethyl- (24) and 2-n-propylthiazolidine (25) were identified and found to possess weak mutagenic activity. In an aqueous fraction, 2-(1,2,3,4,5-pentahydroxy)-n-pentylthiazolidine (26) was isolated and determined to possess some mutagenic activity. Omura *et al.* (1983) investigated the isolation of mutagens in the Maillard reaction of glucose and cysteine, in which a dialyzed sample from the reaction was subjected to GC/MS and the major component in the extract was identified as 2-methylthiazolidine.

22　　23　　24　　25　　26　　27a: R =H
　　　　　　　　　　　　　　　　　　27b: R = alkyl

Thiazolidines can react with nitrite-rich foods such as cured meats to form mutagenic or carcinogenic *N*-nitroso-2-alkylthiazolidines (27, Umano *et al.*, 1984). Sakaguchi and Shibamoto (1979) isolated *N*-nitroso-2-methylthiazolidine as a major volatile product from a cysteamine–acetaldehyde–nitrite model system under simulated cooking conditions. Mihara and Shibamoto (1980) identified *N*-nitroso-2-methylthiazolidine and *N*-nitroso-2-ethylthiazolidine in a reaction mixture obtained from a cysteamine–glucose–nitrite model system. Nitrosothiazolidines have been isolated in cured meat products such as fried bacon, bologna, ham, hot dogs and pepperoni at levels ranging from 1.7 to 19.0 ppb (Loury *et al.*, 1984). *N*-Nitrosothiazolidine (27a) and its nitroso-2-alkyl derivatives (27b) were found to have stronger mutagenic activities than their thiazolidine counterparts in *S. typhimurium* strain TA100 without S9 activation (Mihara and Shibamoto, 1980; Umano *et al.*, 1984). The mutagenic activity of the unsubstituted parent nitrosamine and its 2-alkyl derivatives decreases in the following order: unsubstituted > isopropyl > propyl > ethyl > butyl > isobutyl > methyl.

IMIDAZOLES

Imidazoles have been found in large quantities in the Maillard reaction between L-rhamnose and ammonia (Shibamoto and Bernhard, 1980). Voogd *et al.* (1979) investigated the mutagenic activities of imidazoles and nitroimidazoles and found that 31 nitroimidazoles and imidazoles without nitro groups were mutagenic. However, alkylimidazoles (1-methyl- (**28**), 1,2-dimethyl- (**29**), 2-methyl- (**30**), 1-ethyl- (**31**), 4-methyl- (**32**) and 4,5-dimethylimidazole (**33**)) exhibited no mutagenicity toward *Salmonella typhimurium* strain TA100 (Shibamoto, 1982). Jones and Weisburger (1985) identified a class of mutagenic imidazole compounds, aminomethylimidazole-4-ones, formed from the heated reaction of acetaldehyde, creatinine and threonine. The products, 2-amino-1-methyl-5-propylideneimidazol-4-one (**34**, AMPI) and 2-amino-5-ethylidene-1-methylimidazol-4-one (**35**, AEMI), were isolated, characterized and found to be mutagenic with Ames tester strains TA98, TA100 and TA1538 with S9 activation.

28   29   30   31   32   33

34   35

PYRAZINES

Pyrazine formation in browning systems is related to color formation: the color of the reaction becomes darker as the reaction progresses, and as pyrazine products increase, the color of the mixture changes from colorless to yellow, then brown and finally dark brown (Shibamoto and Bernhard, 1978). General correlations have also been observed between mutagenicity, pyrazine formation and pH. However, as mentioned earlier, Spingarn and Garvie (1979) reported that alkylpyrazines were nonmutagenic in the *Salmonella*/microsomal assay. Stich *et al.* (1980) showed that four alkylpyrazines, 2-methyl- (**36**), 2-ethyl- (**37**), 2,5-dimethyl- (**38**) and 2,6-dimethylpyrazine (**39**), did not exhibit mutagenicity toward *S. typhimurium* strains TA98, TA1537 and TA100, with or without microsomal activation; however, these compounds did respond to

Saccharomyces cerevisiae strain D5 and induced an increase in frequency of chromosomal aberrations in Chinese hamster ovary cells. Other individual pyrazines have been tested for mutagenicity. Shibamoto (1980) determined that tricyclic pyrazines (1,5 **(40)** or 7-dimethyl-2,3,6,7-tetrahydro-1*H*,5*H*-biscyclo-pentapyrazine **(41)**) isolated from a cyclotene/ammonia browning system showed mutagenicity toward *S. typhimurium* strain TA98 and TA1536 without S9 activation. These mutagenic polycyclic pyrazines were the first isolated from aqueous reaction mixtures but have not yet been identified in foods (Shibamoto, 1980).

| 36 | 37 | 38 | 39 |

| *trans* | *cis* | *trans* | *cis* |
| 40 | | 41 | |

FORMATION OF HETEROCYCLIC AROMATIC AMINES

There are four classes of mutagenic heterocyclic amines present in cooked meats: pyrido-imidazoles or -indoles, quinolines, quinoxalines and pyridines (Skog, 1993; Overvik *et al.*, 1993). The pyrido-imidazoles and -indoles shown in Table 7.3 have been identified by pyrolyzing amino acids such as tryptophan, glutamic acid, lysine, phenylalanine, creatinine, and ornithine. The most important factors in the formation of these mutagens are the cooking temperature and time. Overvik and Gustafsson (1990) determined that the mutagenicity of the food increased 5-fold when the pan temperature was increased from 200° to 300 °C. In high-temperature cooking processes such as broiling and grilling, mutagenic pyrolysates from amino acids are formed. Sugimura and colleagues (1977, 1986) reported mutagenic nitrogen containing heterocyclic compounds from pyrolyzed amino acid and protein model systems (550 °C) and high-temperature broiling of chicken and mackerel. Sugimura *et al.* (1977) and Yamamoto *et al.* (1978) isolated 3-amino-1,4-dimethyl-5*H*-pyrido[4,3-*b*]indole (Trp-P-1) and 3-amino-1-methyl-5*H*-pyrido[4,3-*b*]indole (Trp-P-2), and 2-amino-6-methyldipyrido[1,2-*a*: 3′,2′-*d*]imidazole (Glu-P-1) and 2-aminodipyrido[1,2-a:3′,2′*d*]imidazole (Glu-P-2) from the pyrolysates of

Table 7.3. Nomenclature and structure of pyridoimidazole and pyridoindole mutagens formed from amino acid or protein pyrolysates

Mutagen	Abbreviation	Structure
3-Amino-1,4-dimethyl-5*H*-pyrido[4,3-*b*]indole	Trp-P-1	
3-Amino-1-methyl-5*H*-pyrido[4,3-*b*]indole	Trp-P-2	
2-Amino-6-methyldipyrido-[1,2-*a*: 3′,2′-*d*]imidazole	Glu-P-1	
2-Aminodipyrido-[1,2-*a*:3′,2′-*d*]imidazole	Glu-P-2	
3,4-Cyclopentenopyrido-[3,2-*a*]carbazole	Lys-P-1	
4-Amino-6-methyl-1*H*-2,5,10,10-*b*-tetraazafluoranthene	Orn-P-1	
2-Amino-5-phenylpyridine	Phe-P-1	
2-Amino-9*H*-pyrido[2,3-*b*]indole	AαC	
2-Amino-3-methyl-9*H*-pyrido[2,3-*b*]indole	MeAαC	
4-Amino-1,6-dimethyl-2-methylamino-1*H*,6*H*-pyrrolo-[3,4-*f*]benzimidazole-5,7-dione	Cre-P-1	

Table 7.4. Nomenclature and structure of imidazoquinoline and imidazoquinoxaline mutagens

Mutagen	Abbreviation	Structure
2-Amino-3-methylimidazo-[4,5-*f*]quinoline	IQ	
2-Amino-3,4-dimethylimidazo-[4,5-*f*]quinoline	MeIQ	
2-Amino-3-methylimidazo-[4,5-*f*]quinoxaline	IQx	
2-Amino-3,8-dimethylimidazo-[4,5-*f*]quinoxaline	MeIQx	
2-Amino-3,4-dimethylimidazo-[4,5-*f*]quinoxaline	4-MeIQx	
2-Amino-3,4,8-trimethylimidazo-[4,5-*f*]quinoxaline	4,8-DiMeIQx	
2-Amino-3,7,8-trimethylimidazo-[4,5-*f*]quinoxaline	7,8-DiMeIQx	

Table 7.5. Nomenclature and structure of imidazopyridine mutagens

Mutagen	Abbreviation	Structure
2-Amino-1-methyl-6-phenylimidazo[4,5-*b*]pyridine	PhIP	
2-Amino-1,6-dimethylimidazopyridine	DMIP	
2-Amino-n,n,n-trimethyl-imidazopyridine	TMIP	
Methylimidazofuropyridine or 2-amino-(1 or 3),6-dimethylfuro[2,3(or 3,2)-*e*]-imidazo[4,5-*b*]pyridine	MeIFP	

tryptophan and glutamate, respectively. Amino-α-carboline (AαC) and methylamino-α-carboline (MeAαC) were isolated from soybean globulin pyrolysates (Yoshida *et al.*, 1978). These compounds have also been isolated in high-temperature cooked foods such as broiled beef (Trp-P-1, Trp-P-2, AαC), fried ground beef (Trp-P-1, Trp-P-2), broiled chicken (Trp-P-1, Trp-P-2, AαC) and broiled mutton (Trp-P-2, AαC, MeAαC) (Sugimura *et al.*, 1993). In these studies, the yield of the pyrolysates were correlated with the amino acid content in the food (Sugimura, 1986).

In cooked muscle foods, creatine and creatine phosphate participate in the formation of carcinogenic and mutagenic heterocyclic aromatic amines. The structures and nomenclature of these compounds are shown in Tables 7.4 and 7.5 and include imidazoquinolines such as 2-amino-3-methylimidazo[4,5-*f*]quinoline (IQ) and 2-amino-3,4-dimethylimidazo[4,5-*f*]quinoline (MeIQ); imidazoquinoxalines such as 2-amino-3,8-dimethylimidazo[4,5-*f*]quinoxaline (MeIQx) and its isomers 2-amino-3,4-dimethylimidazo[4,5-*f*]-quinoxaline (4-MeIQx) and 2-amino-3,4,8-trimethylimidazo[4,5-*f*]quinoxaline (4,8-DiMeIQx); and imidazopyridines such as 2-amino-1-methyl-6-phenyl-imidazo[4,5-*b*]pyridine (PhIP).

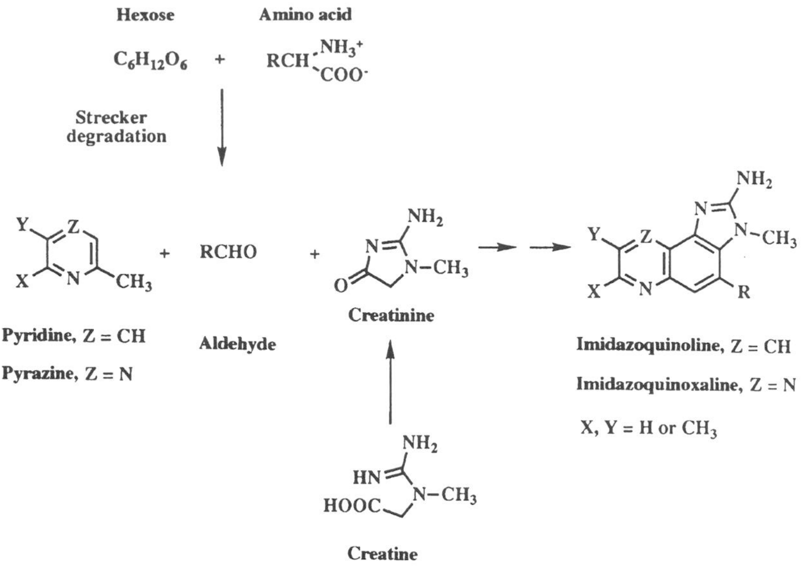

Figure 7.2. Formation of imidazoquinoline and imidazoquinoxaline compounds from amino acid and sugar precursors. (Adapted from Skog, 1993, Jagerstad and Skog, 1983, and O'Brien and Morrissey, 1989)

The formation of these heterocyclic aromatic amines is a result of the heat treatment that causes cyclization of creatine to creatinine to form the imidazole moeity. The remaining moeities of the structure arise from pyridines and pyrazines formed through the Strecker degradation of amino acids and breakdown products of α-dicarbonyl products formed by the Maillard reaction. The reaction of creatinine, amino acid and sugar to form IQ and IQx compounds is shown in Figure 7.2. The aldol condensation is also involved in linking the two groups through a Strecker aldehyde or Schiff base (Skog, 1993). Another hypothesis to IQ formation involves the condensation of aldehydes with creatinine and then condensation with a pyrazine or pyridine (Jagerstad and Skog, 1991). The Strecker degradation, as shown in Figure 7.3, is an essential part of the Maillard reaction which involves the interaction of α-dicarbonyl compounds and α-amino acids. The resulting carboxyaldehydes are created under heated conditions and are degraded into aldehydes, acids, CO_2, pyrazines and other sugar fragmentation products. The mechanisms of IQ and IQx formation were suggested by Jagerstad *et al.* (1983), whose work demonstrated that the Maillard reaction is important in the formation of these mutagens (Skog and Jagerstad, 1993).

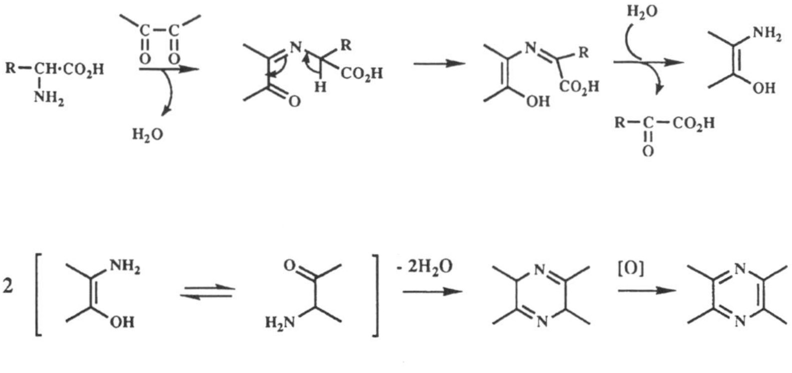

Figure 7.3. Strecker degradation of amino acids and Maillard reaction intermediates to form heterocyclic compounds

The factors involved in the formation of these IQ compounds in model systems are the creatine, amino acid and sugar content, and temperature (Johansson and Jagerstad, 1993; Skog, 1993; Knize *et al.*, 1994b). In model systems, the mutagenic activity was present in the temperature range of 150–200 °C (Skog, 1993). Mutagenicity was not detected in a glycine–creatinine–glucose system below 140 °C for 15 min, but it was detected when the temperatures were elevated to 160° and above. Creatine is essential for mutagen formation because it was shown that low creatine, high protein foods contained low levels of mutagens after cooking (Laser-Reutersward *et al.*, 1987; Overvik *et al.*, 1993). The addition of different types and amounts of amino acids affect mutagen formation (Overvik *et al.*, 1989; Skog, 1993). Jagerstad *et al.* (1983) found that IQ and MeIQ are the significant products formed from the precursors glycine and alanine, respectively, with creatinine and a carbohydrate in model systems. In model systems with creatinine and glucose, the presence of threonine, glycine and lysine produced the highest mutagenic activities, while tryptophan and proline reduced the formation of mutagens. The addition of sugars such as glucose, fructose, ribose, galactose, arabinose and erythrose in model and real food systems increases mutagen formation. Jagerstad *et al.* (1983) showed that the mutagenic activity of fried lean beef containing varying amounts of glucose increased with glucose content. Skog and Jagerstad (1993) incorporated ^{14}C-labeled glucose in a mixture of creatinine, threonine and glucose and clearly demonstrated that glucose is an important precursor in the formation of MeIQx and 4,8-DiMeIQx. It was determined that the C-4 benzene carbon of the IQ compounds originated from the α-carbon of the amino acid, whereas the C-5 carbon and the pyridine/pyrazine carbons originated from the sugar.

FOOD SYSTEMS ASSOCIATED WITH
THE MAILLARD REACTION

The methods to identify and quantitate cooked food mutagens face many problems such as time-consuming analytical procedures, requirements of large amounts of samples and difficulties in quantitation (Nishimura, 1986). Isolation and characterization of mutagens in food systems were initiated in the late 1970s when Kasai *et al.* (1980, 1981) identified three potent mutagens from broiled sardines and beef. Advances in column and detection technology and high-performance liquid chromatography/mass spectrometry (HPLC/MS) in conjunction with nuclear magnetic resonance (NMR) and ultraviolet (UV) methods stimulated the isolation and identification of mutagens, such as heterocyclic aromatic amines from model and real food samples (Nishimura, 1986; Jagerstad *et al.*, 1991). Detection methods for HPLC such as electrochemical, photodiode UV array and on-line scintillation detection were used to analyze IQ, MeIQ and MeIQx in beef extracts. The development of new techniques and improved analytical strategies have been effective in identifying many of these mutagens (Felton *et al.*, 1986). For instance, Gross (1990) developed an effective tandem solid-phase extraction method using diatomaceous earth and copper phthalocyanine-derivatized Sephasorb cartridges to extract mutagenic heterocyclic aromatic amines from meat products. In early analytical developments, Jagerstad *et al.* (1983) and Nyhammar *et al.* (1986) separated mutagens formed in model systems and cooked meats by C-18 reverse-phase HPLC and ion-exchange chromatography, identified the mutagens by ^{1}H-NMR and MS, and tested their mutagenic activities by the *Salmonella*/microsomal assay. Nishimura (1986) indicated that the superior sensitivity and selectivity of gas chromatography/mass spectrometry (GC/MS) methods using isotope-labeled internal standards could be effective for the analysis of mutagenic heterocyclic aromatic amines. IQ and MeIQ were extracted from broiled sardines and analyzed by GC/MS. However, only 0.1–0.01% of the total mutagen was quantitatively determined due to column deterioration by the sample. Edmonds *et al.* (1986) have demonstrated the use of HPLC/MS to analyze heterocyclic aromatic mutagens in cooked meats in the parts per billion concentration range. They were able to detect concentration level ranges of 0.2–0.4 and 0.4–0.9 μg/kg for IQ and MeIQ, respectively, in broiled salmon. The LC/MS methods demonstrate detection selectivity and sensitivity; improved quantitative analysis can be further achieved by the use of deuterated internal standards. Thiebaud *et al.* (1994) have recently used supercritical fluid extraction, vapor trap techniques and GC/MS to extract and analyze heterocyclic amines from fumes isolated from fried beef patties. The major components in the meat and fume condensates were PhIP and AαC, respectively. MeIQx and DiMeIQx were detected, but IQ and other pyrolysates were not. In addition to the identification of heterocyclic aromatic amines, GC/MS analysis identified a variety of ketones, aldehydes and phenols in the fume condensates.

COFFEE

According to Nagao *et al.* (1986), one cup of coffee contains mutagens that produce $5 \times 10^4 - 10^5$ revertants in *S. typhimurium* strain TA100 with S9 activation. Nagao *et al.* (1983, 1986), Aeschbacher and Wurzner (1980) and Friederich *et al.* (1985) demonstrated that instant, regular, caffeine-free and freshly brewed coffees were mutagenic in *S. typhimurium* strains TA100, TA102 and TA104, *E. coli* WP2*uvrA*/pKM101 in the absence of S9 microsomal activation and diphtheria toxin-resistant mutation in Chinese hamster lung cells *in vitro*. The formation of mutagens was attributed to the roasting process of the beans, since coffee prepared from green beans did not induce any mutagenic activity (Albertini *et al.*, 1985). The mutagens in coffee were identified to be dicarbonyl compounds such as methyl glyoxal, diacetyl and glyoxal. Fujita *et al.* (1985) suggested that a possible synergistic effect between the oxidant hydrogen peroxide and methyl glyoxal account for the total mutagenicity in coffee. However, Ariza *et al.* (1988) attributed 40–60% of the mutagenicity to hydrogen peroxide since the addition of the antioxidant enzyme catalase abolished more than 95% of the mutagenicity. In these studies, the more sensitive L-arabinose resistance forward mutation assay with *S. typhimurium* without S9 activation was used rather than the usual histidine reverse mutation assay. Other investigators have identified that the heterocyclic aromatic amine, MeIQ, is also present in coffee beans (Kikugawa *et al.*, 1989; Kato *et al.*, 1989; Kato *et al.*, 1991). Kato *et al.* (1994) have identified another class of mutagens in coffee which they believed is derived from the Maillard reaction. However, these mutagenic Maillard reaction products have not been identified.

MILK

The presence of reducing sugars and amino groups in milk has led investigators to research the formation of mutagens in commercially heat-sterilized milk. Green *et al.* (1980) discovered that commercially sterilized milk was mutagenic in *S. thyphimurium* strains TA98 and TA100 with S9 activation. Sekizawa and Shibamoto (1986) studied heat-processed milk samples treated by heat sterilization and pasteurization. Dichloromethane extracts of the milk heated at 100, 135 and 150 °C for 5 h exhibited no mutagenicity in *S. typhimurium* strains TA98 and TA100 with and without S9 activation. Berg *et al.* (1990) also confirmed that heated skim or sterilized milk did not possess mutagenic activity. It is suggested that mutagenic formation is suppressed by interactions with various milk constituents such as casein.

STARCH-CONTAINING FOODS

Pariza *et al.* (1979) investigated the mutagenic activities of bakery and cereal products using *S. typhimurium* strain TA98 with S9 activation. Crackers, corn flakes, rice cereal and bread crusts showed low levels of mutagenicity, while white bread crumbs, toast and cookies all showed marginal levels of mutagenic activity. Spingarn *et al.* (1980) tested several starchy foods such as fried potatoes, toasted white and dark breads and pancakes, and detected mutagenic activity on *S. typhimurium* strains TA98 and TA100 with S9 activation. The mutagenicity of toasted pumpernickel bread showed a higher activity than toasted white bread. However, the number of revertants in one slice of toasted pumpernickel is only about 5% of that found in a cooked beef patty. The mutagenic activity of starch-containing foods of low protein and high carbohydrate content was attributed to the Maillard reaction. The sugar and starch breakdown during the heating process forms reactive and unsaturated aldehydes and ketones, while amino acids and amines are degraded by heat to form Amadori compounds with carbonyls. These fragments and byproducts can react, cyclize and dehydrate to form a variety of heteroaromatic structures. Friedman *et al.* (1990b) studied the mutagen formation in heated wheat gluten, carbohydrates and gluten/carbohydrate blends using *Salmonella* strains TA98, TA100, TA102 and TA1537 with and without S9 activation. They found high mutagenicity in heated gluten using the tester strain TA98 with S9 activation but discovered weak mutagenic responses in TA100 and TA102 with and without S9 mix. The baked carbohydrates were moderately mutagenic in the tester strain TA98 with S9 activation, but weak without S9 activation in the tester strains TA100, TA102 and TA1537. Heated blends were not found to be mutagenic. Knize *et al.* (1994a) investigated the mutagenic activity in gluten, wheat gluten, corn meal, garbanzo flour, teff flour, rice flour, rye flour and wheat flour heated at 210 °C and found that garbanzo and wheat flour and wheat gluten had higher mutagenicities, while rice and rye flours did not produce any mutagenic activities in *S. typhimurium* strain TA98 with S9 activation. Increases in the heating time of the flours did result in an increase of mutagenicity. Among the toasted foods, products made from wheat flour had the higher mutagenic activity than products made with corn or rice flours. Heterocyclic aromatic amines found in the extracts of breadsticks, heated gluten and grain beverages were MeIQx, DiMeIQx, Trp-P-2, Trp-P-1, AαC and PhIP. However, meat-substitute grain patties (gluten-based patties made from tofu, falafel and tempeh burger) only possessed approximately 10% of the mutagenicity found in cooked ground beef.

FRUIT JUICES AND DRIED FRUITS

The drying and curing of fruits can induce chemical changes that include Maillard browning, enzymatic browning and caramelization. Stich *et al.*

(1981a, 1981b) investigated the clastogenic activities of dried fruits in Chinese hamster ovary cells with S9 activation. Black and golden raisins, prunes, dates, bananas, figs and apricots were shown to possess strong chromosome-damaging capacities.

Ekasari *et al.* (1986) studied and found mutagenic activity in fresh orange juice heated at 93 °C for 30 min in *S. typhimurium* strain TA100. Fresh-pressed orange juice possessed no mutagenic properties, the mutagenicity being induced by the heat treatment. These investigators proposed that the mutagenic response is due to Maillard browning. In later studies, Ekasari *et al.* (1990) attempted to characterize the mutagenic compounds in the heated orange juice using ion-exchange chromatography and solvent extraction. Their results showed that these mutagens were neutral, polar and nonvolatile compounds of molecular weights less than 700 daltons. Analysis by fast atom bombardment mass spectrometry was used to determine the molecular weights of these mutagens at 162, 180, 254, 288, 342 and 540 daltons (Ekasari *et al.*, 1993); the elemental compositions of some of these compounds were determined to be $C_6H_{12}O_6$, $C_9H_{18}O_{11}$, $C_{11}H_{20}O_{13}$ and $C_{11}H_{22}O_{15}$. In another study, Friedman *et al.* (1990a) studied the mutagenic responses of fresh and heated orange, apple, grape and pear juices in *S. typhimurium* strains TA98, TA100, TA102 and TA2637 with and without S9 activation. Results show that fresh orange juice yielded revertant frequencies 2–3 times greater than the water controls, but the mutagenic levels of the heated juices were the same as the fresh juices.

COOKED MEATS

Kasai *et al.* (1980, 1981) first isolated IQ and MeIQ from broiled sardines and MeIQx from fried beef. Nishimura (1986) isolated from broiled sardines a variety of mutagens such as Trp-P-1, Trp-P-2, Glu-P-1, Glu-P-2, Lys-P-1, AαC, MeAαC, MeIQ and IQ. In fried beef, Felton *et al.* (1986) quantitated levels of IQ, IQx and IP compounds and found that the majority of the mutagenic activity was attributed to MeIQx, DiMeIQx, TMIP and PhIP, with smaller contributions from IQ, MeIQ and three unidentified polar mutagens. Cooked meats contain roughly 1–70 ng/g of heterocyclic amines, and several different heterocyclic aromatic amines have been isolated, identified and quantitated in cooked meat products, as shown in Table 7.6. In addition, meat mutagens have been isolated from the crust of broiled, fried and baked meats such as beef, pork, ham, bacon, chicken and lamb, as well as heat-treated meat extracts such as gravies and bouillons (Jagerstad and Skog, 1991).

The relationships between mutagen formation, cooking time and temperature of cooked foods have shown that frying, grilling and broiling are the most effective methods in mutagen formation. Barrington *et al.* (1990) examined mutagen formation in lamb and beef using common household cooking

Table 7.6. Imidazoquinoline (IQ), imidazoquinoxaline (IQx) and imidazopyridine (IP) compounds present in cooked meats. (Adapted from Skog, 1993)

Food	Mutagens present
Broiled beef	IQ, MeIQx, PhIP
Broiled ground beef	IQ
Fried ground beef	IQ, MeIQ, MeIQx, 4,8-DiMeIQx, PhIP, TMIP
Broiled sardine	IQ, MeIQ
Broiled salmon	IQ, MeIQ, MeIQx, PhIP
Fried fish	IQ, MeIQ, 4,8-DiMeIQx, PhIP
Beef extract	IQ, MeIQx, 4,8-DiMeIQx, PhIP
Fried beef	MeIQx, 4,8-DiMeIQx, PhIP
Fried hamburger	MeIQx, 4,8-DiMeIQx
Broiled chicken	MeIQx, 4,8-DiMeIQx, PhIP
Broiled mutton	MeIQx, 4,8-DiMeIQx
Smoked fish	MeIQx

methods such as grilling, frying, roasting, stewing, boiling and microwave-cooked lamb and beef contained little or no mutagenicity in *S. typhimurium* strain TA1538 with S9 activation. However, fried and grilled meats had significantly higher levels of mutagenicity, which was attributed to high surface temperatures and the use of butter in grilling and frying techniques. Yoshida *et al.* (1986) showed that high-temperature processes such as grilling form the amino-α-carbolines, AαC, as well as Trp-P-2 in grilled beef, chicken, mushrooms and onions. Minimum cooking temperatures such as microwave treatment or stewing (low-temperature simmering) produce negligible amounts of mutagens in meats, whereas fried and broiled meats can contain up to several micrograms (Barnes *et al.*, 1983). However, Taylor *et al.* (1986) and Lee *et al.* (1994b) were able to find IQ, MeIQ, and Trp-P-2 in boiled beef juice and IQ, MeIQ, MeIQx and possible diMeIQx isomers in boiled pork juice, respectively. In the boiled pork study, the amounts of IQ mutagens were actually higher than those found in broiled beef and fried ground beef.

A comprehensive study to identify the genotoxic risks of IQ and MeIQx in cooked meat products was performed by Loprieno *et al.* (1991). Their work involved the identification and quantification of IQx and MeIQx from a cooked veal extract and genotoxicity and mutagenicity studies using the *Salmonella*/Ames assay, chromosomal aberration assays in Chinese hamster ovary cell line and cultured human lymphocytes, toxicokinetic and distribution studies in laboratory mice and DNA binding studies. In their work, the mutagens induced gene mutation in *Salmonella*, but not in Chinese hamster cells, and IQ induced chromosomal aberrations in Chinese hamster ovary cells and human lymphocytes. Both mutagens were found to bind to DNA but were negative for micronuclei induction in laboratory mice. However, when the collected data were compared to other studies, the investigators concluded that a relationship existed between mutagenesis, carcinogenesis and genotoxicity with dietary meat intake and everyday cooking practices.

Fat drippings and grill residue scrapings from cooked meats used as bases for gravies and sauces and dietary habits have a strong impact of heterocyclic aromatic amine exposure. Gross *et al.* (1993) measured the amounts of heterocyclic aromatic amines (HAAs) in grilled meat patties and found levels of MeIQx and PhIP ranging from 0.8 to 3.2 ppb. Bacon contained PhIP and MeIQx levels ranging from 0.1 to 52 and 0.9 to 18 ppb, respectively. Although the amounts of HAAs found in cooked foods are low, Gross *et al.* (1993) believed that the epidemiological and exposure data support a plausible role of these compounds in human carcinogenesis, particularly in relation between colorectal cancer and meat consumption. Therefore, meat intake combined with frequent consumptions of meat-based gravies and popular grilled cooking techniques can substantially increase the risk of colorectal cancer.

CONCLUSION

The Maillard reaction is responsible for the formation of mutagenic compounds formed in several degradation pathways or by Maillard reaction intermediates combining with other chemical constituents in foods. The diversity of the mutagens ranges from simple dicarbonyl compounds and heterocyclic volatiles to heterocyclic aromatic amines. The advanced analytical developments and genotoxic testing techniques used to identify and quantify such compounds in foods and to assess their mutagenicity have provided information to establish relationships between dietary intake and carcinogenesis. Research in these areas is improving and continues to be assessed.

REFERENCES

Aeaschbacher, H. U., and Wurzner, H. P. (1980). An evaluation of instant and regular coffee in the Ames mutagenicity test, *Toxicol. Lett.*, **5**(2), 139–45.

Albertini, S., Friederich, U., Schlatter, C., and Wurgler, F. E. (1985). The influence of roasting procedure on the formation of mutagenic compounds in coffee, *Food Chem. Toxicol.*, **23**(6), 593–7.

Ames, B. N., McCann, J., and Yamasaki, E. (1975). Methods for detecting carcinogens and mutagens with the *Salmonella*/mammalian-microsome mutagenicity test. *Mutation Res.*, **31**, 347–64.

Anderson, D. (1988). Genetic toxicology. In D. Anderson and D. M. Conning (eds.), *Experimental Toxicology: The Basic Principles*, The Royal Society of Chemistry, London, pp. 242–86.

Ariza, R. R., Dorado, G., Barbancho, M., and Pueyo, C. (1988). Study of the causes of direct-acting mutagenicity in coffee and tea using the Ara test in *Salmonella typhimurium*, *Mutation Res.*, **201**, 89–96.

Barnes, W., Spingarn, N. E., Garvie-Gould, C., Vuolo, L. L., Wang, Y. Y., and Weisburger, J. H. (1983). Mutagens in cooked foods: possible consequences of the Maillard reaction. In G. R. Waller and M. S. Feather (eds.), *The Maillard Reaction in Foods and Nutrition*, American Chemistry Society, Washington, D.C., pp. 486–505.

Barrington, P. J., Baker, R. S. U., Truswell, A. S., Bonin, A. M., Ryan, A. J. and Paulin, A. P. (1990). Mutagenicity of basic fractions derived from lamb and beef cooked by common household methods, *Food Chem. Toxicol.*, **28**(3), 141–6.

Berg, H. E., van Boekel, M. A. J. S., and Jongen, W. M. F. (1990). Heating milk: a study on mutagenicity, *J. Food Sci.*, **55**(4), 1000–4, 1017.

Bjeldanes, L. F. and Chew, H. (1979). Mutagenicity of 1,2-dicarbonyl compounds: maltol, kojic acid, diacetyl and related substances. *Mutation Res.*, **67**, 367–71.

Chan, R. I. M., Stich, H. F., Rosin, M. P., and Powrie, W. D. (1982). Antimutagenic activity of browning reaction products, *Cancer Lett.*, **15**, 27–33.

Edmonds, C. G., Sethi, S. K., Yamaizumi, Z., Kasai, H., Nishimura, S., and McCloskey, J. A. (1986). Analysis of mutagens from cooked foods by directly combined liquid chromatography–mass spectrometry, *Environ. Health Perspect.*, **67**, 35–40.

Ekasari, I., Jongen, W. M. F., and Pilnik, W. (1986). Use of a bacterial mutagenicity assay as a rapid method for the detection of early stage of Maillard reactions in orange juices, *Food Chem.*, **21**, 125–31.

Ekasari, I., Berg, H. E., Jongen, W. M. F., and Pilnik, W. (1990). Characterization of mutagenic compound(s) in heated orange juice, *Food Chem.*, **36**, 11–18.

Ekasari, I., Fokkens, R. H., Bonestroo, M. H., Schols, H. A., Nibbering, N. M. M., and Pilnik, W. (1993). Characterization of mutagenic compounds in heated orange juice by UV and mass spectra, *Food Chem.*, **46**, 77–9.

Felton, J. S., Knize, M. G., Shen, N. H., Andresen, B. D., Bjeldanes, L. F., and Hatch, F. T. (1986). Identification of the mutagens in cooked beef, *Environ. Health Perspect.*, **67**, 17–24.

Friedrich, U., Hann, D., Albertini, S., Schlatter, C., and Wurgler, F. E. (1985). Mutagenicity studies on coffee. The influence of different factors on the mutagenic activity in the *Salmonella*/mammalian microsomal assay, *Mutation Res.*, **156**(1–2), 39–52.

Friedman, M., Wilson, R. E., and Ziderman, I. I. (1990a). Effect of heating of mutagenicity of fruit juices in the Ames test. *J. Agric. Food Chem.*, **38**, 740–3.

Friedman, M., Wilson, R. E., and Ziderman, I. I. (1990b). Mutagen formation in a heated wheat gluten, carbohydrate and gluten/carbohydrate blends, *J. Agric. Food Chem.*, **38**, 1019–28.

Fujita, Y., Wakabayashi, K., Nagao, M., and Sugimura, T. (1985). Characteristics of major mutagenicity of instant coffee, *Mutation Res.*, **142**, 145–8.

Gazzani, G., Vagnarelli, P., Cuzzoni, M. T., and Mazza, P. G. (1987). Mutagenic activity of the Maillard reaction products of ribose with different amino acids, *J. Food Sci.*, **52**(3), 757–60.

Green, M., Ben-Hur, E., Riklis, E., Gordon, S., and Rosenthal, I. (1980). Application of mutagenicity test for milk, *J. Dairy Sci.*, **63**, 358.

Gross, G. A. (1990). Simple methods for quantifying mutagenic heterocyclic aromatic amines in food products, *Carcinogenesis*, **11**(9), 1597–603.

Gross, G. A., Turesky, R. J., Fay, L. B., Stillwell, W. G., Skipper, P. L., and Tannenbaum, S. R. (1993). Heterocyclic aromatic amine formation in grilled bacon, beef and fish and in grill scrapings, *Carcinongenesis*, **14**(11), 2313–18.

Hiramoto, K., Kido, K., and Kikugawa, K. (1994). DNA breaking by Maillard products of glucose–amino acid mixtures formed in aqueous systems, *J. Agric. Food Chem.*, **42**, 689–94.

Hodge, J. E. (1953). Chemistry of browning reactions in model systems, *J. Agric. Food Chem.*, **1**, 928–43.

Jagerstad, M., and Skog, K. (1991). Formation of meat mutagens. In M. Friedman (ed.), *Nutritional and Toxicological Consequences of Food Processing*, Plenum Press, New York, pp. 83–105.

Jagerstad, M., Laser-Reutersward, A., Oste, R., and Dahlquist, A. (1983). Creatinine and Maillard reaction products as precursors of mutagenic compounds formed in fried beef. In G. R. Wallen and M. S. Feather (eds.), *The Maillard Reaction in Foods and Nutrition*, American Chemical Society, Washington D.C., pp. 507–19.

Jagerstad, M., Skog, K., Grivas, S., and Olsson, K. (1991). Formation of heterocyclic amines using model systems. *Mutation Res.*, **259**, 219–33.

Johansson, M., and Jagerstad, M. (1993). Influence of oxidized deep-frying fat and iron on the formation of food mutagens in a model system, *Food Chem. Toxicol.*, **31**(12), 971–9.

Jones, R. C., and Weisburger, J. H. (1989). Characterization of aminoalkylimidazol-4-one mutagens from liquid reflux models, *Mutation Res.*, **222**, 43–51.

Kasai, H., Yamaizumi, Z., Wakabayashi, K., Nagao, M., Sugimura, T., Yokoyama, S., Miyazawa, T., and Nishimuram, S. (1980). Structure of a potent mutagen isolated from broiled fish, *Chem. Lett.*, 1391–4.

Kasai, H., Yamaizumi, Z., Shiomi, T., Yokoyama, S., Miyazawa, T., Wakabayashi, K., Nagao, M., Sugimura, T., and Nishimura, S. (1981). Structure of a potent mutagen isolated from fried beef, *Chem. Lett.*, 485–8.

Kato, T., Takahashi, S., and Kikugawa, K. (1991). Loss of heterocyclic amine mutagens by insoluble hemicellulose fiber and high-molecular-weight soluble phenophenolics of coffee, *Mutation Res.*, **246**(1), 165–78.

Kato, T., Hiramoto, K., and Kikugawa, K. (1994). Possible occurrence of new mutagens with the DNA breaking activity in coffee, *Mutation Res.*, **306**, 9–17.

Kikugawa, K., Kato, T., and Takahashi, S. (1989). Possible presence of 2-amino-3,4-dimethylimidazo[4,5-*f*]quinoline and other heterocyclic amine-like mutagens in roasted coffee beans, *J. Agric. Food Chem.*, **37**(4), 881–6.

Knize, M. G., Roper, M., Shen, N. H., and Felton, J. S. (1990). Proposed structures for an amino-dimethylimidazofuropyridine mutagen in cooked meats, *Carcinogenesis*, **11**(12), 2259–62.

Knize, M. G., Cunningham, P. L., Griffin, E. A., Jones, A. L., and Felton, J. S. (1994a). Characterization of mutagenic activity in cooked-grain-food products, *Food Chem. Toxicol.*, **32**(1), 15–21.

Knize, M. G., Dolbeare, F. A., Carroll, K. C., Moore, D. H., and Felton, J. S. (1994b). Effect of cooking time and temperature on the heterocyclic amine content of fried beef patties, *Food Chem. Toxicol.*, **32**(7), 595–603.

Kong, Z. L., Shinohara, K., Mitsuki, M., Murrakami, H., and Omura, H. (1989). Desmutagenicity of furan compounds towards some mutagens, *Agric. Biol. Chem.*, **53**(8), 2073–9.

Laser-Reutersward, A., Skog, K., and Jagerstad, M. (1987). Mutagenicity of pan-fried bovine tissues in relation to their content of creatine, creatinine, monosaccharides and free amino acids, *Food Chem. Toxicol.*, **25**, 755–62.

Lee, H., Bian, S. S., and Chen, Y. L. (1994a). Genotoxicity of 1,3-dithiane and 1,4-dithiane in the CHO/SCE assay and the *Salmonella*/microsomal test, *Mutation Res.*, **321**, 213–18.

Lee, H., Lin, M. Y., and Chan, L. C. (1994b). Formation and identification of carcinogenic heterocyclic aromatic amines in boiled pork juice, *Mutation Res.*, **308**, 77–88.

Lopriento, N., Boncristiani, G., and Lopriento, G. (1991). An experimental approach to identifying the genotoxic risk by cooked meat mutagens. In M. Friedman (ed.), *Nutritional and Toxicological Consequences of Food Processing*, Plenum Press, New York, pp. 115–31.

Loury, D. J., Byard, J. L., and Shibamoto, T. (1984). Genotoxicity of *N*-nitrosothiazolidine in microbial and hepatocellular test systems, *Food Chem. Toxicol.*, **22**(12), 1013–14.

Maga, J. A., and Sizer, C. E. (1973). Pyrazines in foods, *CRC Critical Reviews in Food Technology*, **1973**, 39.

Maron, D. M., and Ames, B. N. (1983). Revised methods for the Salmonella mutagenicity test, *Mutation Res.*, **113**, 173–215.

Mihara, S., and Shibamoto, T. (1980). Mutagenicity of products obtained from cysteamine–glucose browning model systems, *J. Agric. Food Chem.*, **28**, 62–6.

Nagao, M., Sato, S., and Sugimura, T. (1983). Mutagens produced by heating foods. In G. R. Waller and M. S. Feather (eds.), *The Maillard Reaction in Foods and Nutrition*, American Chemical Society, Washington, D. C., pp. 521–36.

Nagao, M., Fujita, Y., Wakabayashi, K., Nukaya, H., Kosuge, T., and Sugimura, T. (1986). Mutagens in coffee and other beverages, *Environ. Health Perspect.*, **67**, 89–91.

Nishimura, S. (1986). Chemistry of mutagens and carcinogens in broiled foods, *Environmental Health Perspectives*, **67**, 11–16.

Nyhammar, T., Grivas, S., Olsson, K., and Jagerstad, M. (1986). Isolation and identification of beef mutagens (IQ compounds) from heated model systems of creatinine, fructose and glycine or alanine. In M. Fujimaki, M. Namiki, and H. Kato (eds.), *Amino-Carbonyl Reactions in Food and Biological Systems*, Kodansha, Ltd, Tokyo, and Elsevier Science Publishers, Amsterdam, The Netherlands, pp. 323–34.

O'Brien, J., and Morrissey, P. A. (1989). Nutritional and toxicological aspects of the Maillard browning reaction in foods, *Critical Reviews in Food Science and Nutrition*, **28**(3), 211–48.

Omura, H., Jahan, N., Shinohara, K., and Murakami, H. (1983). Formation of mutagens by the Maillard Reaction. In G. R. Waller and M. S. Feather (eds.), *The Maillard Reaction in Foods and Nutrition*, American Chemical Society, Washington, D. C., pp. 537–63.

Overvik, E., and Gustafsson, J. A. (1990). Cooked-food mutagens: current knowledge of formation and biological significance, *Mutagenesis*, **5**(5), 437–46.

Overvik, E., Kleman, M., Berg, I., and Gustafson, J. A. (1989). Influence of creatine, amino acids and water on the formation of the mutagenic heterocyclic amines found in cooked meat, *Carcinogenesis* **10**(12), 2293–301.

Overvik, E., Hellmold, H., Kleman, M., and Gustafsson, J.-A. (1993). Formation and toxicity of food pyrolysis mutagens. In D. V. Parke, C. Ioannides, and R. Walker (eds.), *Food, Nutrition and Toxicity*, Smith-Gordon, Great Britain, pp. 277–86.

Pariza, M. W., Ashoor, S. H., and Chu, F. S. (1979). Mutagens in heat-processed meat, bakery and cereal products, *Food and Cosmetic Toxicol.*, **17**, 429–30.

Pintauro, S. J., Page, G. V., Solberg, M., Lee, F. C., and Chichester, C. O. (1980). Absence of mutagenic response from extracts of Maillard browned egg albumin, *J. Food Sci.*, **45**, 1442–3.

Powrie, W. D., Wu, C. H., Rosin, M. P., and Stich, H. F. (1981). Clastogenic and mutagenic activities of Maillard reaction model systems, *J. Food Sci.*, **46**, 1433–8.

Powrie, W. D., Wu, C. H., and Molund, V. P. (1986). Browning reaction systems as sources of mutagens and antimutagens, *Environ. Health Perspect.*, **67**, 47–54.

Rogers, A. M., and Shibamoto, T. (1982). Mutagenicity of the products obtained from heated milk samples, *Food Chem. Toxicol.*, **20**, 259–63.

Sakaguchi, M., and Shibamoto, T. (1979). Isolation of *N*-nitroso-2-methyl-thiazolidine from a cysteamine–acetaldehyde–sodium nitrite model system, *Agric. Biol. Chem.*, **43**, 667–9.

Sekizawa, J., and Shibamoto, T. (1980). Mutagenicity of 2-alkyl-*N*-nitrothiazolidine, *J. Agric. Food Chem.*, **28**, 781–3.

Sekizawa, J., and Shibamoto, T. (1986). *Salmonella*/microsome mutagenicity tests of heat-processed milk samples, *Food Chem. Toxicol.*, **24**(9), 987–8.

Shibamoto, T. (1980). Mutagenicity of 1,5(or 7)-dimethyl-2,3,6,7-tetrahydro-1*H*-bicyclopentapyrazine obtained from a cyclotene/NH_3 browning model system, *J. Agric. Food Chem.*, **28**, 883–4.

Shibamoto, T. (1982). Occurrence of mutagenic products in browning model systems, *Food Technol.*, **1982**, 59–62.

Shibamoto, T. (1983). Heterocyclic compounds in browning and browning/nitrate model systems: occurrence formation mechanisms, flavor characteristics, and mutagenic activity. In G. Charalambous and G. Inglett (eds.), *Instrumental Analysis of Foods*, Vol. 1, Academic Press, New York, pp. 229–78.

Shibamoto, T. (1989). Genotoxicity testing of Maillard reaction products. In J. E. Baynes and V. M. Monnier (eds.), *The Maillard Reaction in Aging, Diabetes and Nutrition*, Alan R. Liss, New York, pp. 359–76.

Shibamoto, T., and Bernhard, R. A. (1978). Formation of heterocyclic compounds from the reaction of L-rhamnose with ammonia, *J. Agric. Food Chem.*, **26**, 183–7.

Shibamoto, T., and Bernhard, R. A. (1980). Heterocyclic compounds found in foods, *J. Agric. Food Chem.*, **28**, 237–43.

Shibamoto, T., Nishimura, O., and Mihara, S. (1981). Mutagenicity of products obtained from a maltol–ammonia browning model system, *J. Agric. Food Chem.*, **29**, 643–6.

Shinohara, K., Wu, R. T., Jahan, N., Tanaka, M., Morinaga, N., Murakami, H., and Omura, H. (1980). Mutagenicity of the browning mixtures by amino-carbonyl reactions on *Salmonella typhimurium* TA100, *Agric. Biol. Chem.*, **44**, 671–5.

Shinohara, K., Kim, E. H., and Omura, H. (1986). Furans as the mutagens formed by amino-carbonyl reactions. In M. Fujimaki, M. Namiki, and H. Kato (eds.), Kodansha, Ltd, Tokyo, and Elsevier Science Publishers, Amsterdam, The Netherlands, pp. 353–62.

Skog, K. (1993). Cooking procedures and food mutagens: a literature review, *Food Chem. Toxicol.*, **31**(9), 655–75.

Skog, K., and Jagerstad, M. (1990). Effects of monosaccharides and disaccharides on the formation of food mutagens in model systems, *Mutation Res.*, **230**(2), 263–76.

Skog, K., and Jagerstad, M. Incorporation of carbon atoms from glucose into the food mutagens MeIQx and 4,8-DiMeIQx using ^{14}C-labelled glucose in a model system, *Carcinogenesis*, **14**(10), 2027–31.

Spingarn, N. E., and Garvie, C. T. (1979). Formation of mutagens in sugar-ammonia model system, *J. Agri. Food Chem.*, **27**(6), 1319–21.

Spingarn, N. E., Slocum, L. A., and Weisburger, J. H. (1980). Formation of mutagens in cooked foods. II. Foods with high starch content, *Cancer Lett.*, **9**, 7–12.

Spingarn, N. E., Garvie-Gould, C. T., and Slocum, L. A. (1983). Formation of mutagens in sugar–amino acid model systems, *J. Agric. Food Chem.*, **31**, 301–4.

Stich, H. F., Stich, W., Rosin, M. P., and Powrie, W. D. Mutagenic activity of pyrazine derivatives: a comparative study with *Salmonella typhimurium*, *Saccharomyces cerevisiae* and Chinese hamster ovary cells, *Food and Cosmetics Toxicol.*, **18**(6), 581–4.

Stich, H. F., Rosin, M. P., Wu, C. H., and Powrie, W. D. (1981a). Clastogenic activity of dried fruits, *Cancer Lett.*, **12**, 1–8.

Stich, H. F., Stich, W., Rosin, M. P., and Powrie, W. D. (1981b). Clastogenic activity of caramel and caramelized sugars, *Mutation Res.*, **91**, 129–35.

Sugimura, T. (1986). Past, present, and future of mutagens in cooked foods, *Environ. Health Perspect.*, **67**, 5–10.

Sugimura, T., Kawachi, T., Nagao, M., Yahagi, T., Sano, Y., Okamoto, T., Shudo, K., Kosuge, T., Tsuji, K., Wakabayashi, K., Iitaka, Y., and Itai, A. (1977). Mutagenic principles in tryptophan and phenylalanine pyrolysis products, *Proc. Japan Academy*, **53B**, 58–61.

Sugimura, T., Wakabayashi, K., Nagao, M., and Esumi, H. (1993). A new class of carcinogens: heterocyclic amines in cooked food. In D. V. Parke, C. Ioannides, and R. Walker (eds.), *Food, Nutrition and Chemical Toxicity*, Smith-Gordon, Great Britain, pp. 275–6.

Taylor, R. T., Fultz, E., and Knize, M. G. (1986). Mutagen formation in model beef supernatant fractions. IV. Properties of the system, *Environ. Health Perspect.*, **67**, 59–74.

Thiebaud, H. P., Knize, M. G., Kuzmicky, P. A., Felton, J. S., and Hseih, D. P. (1994). Mutagenicity and chemical analysis of fumes from cooking meat, *J. Agric. Food Chem.*, **42**, 1502–10.

Toda, H., Sekizawa, J., and Shibamoto, T. (1981). Mutagenicity of the L-rhamnose–ammonia–hydrogen sulfide browning reaction mixture, *J. Agric. Food Chem.*, **29**, 381–4.

Umano, K., Shibamoto, T., Fernando, S. Y., and Wei, C. I. (1984). Mutagenicity of 2-hydroxyalkyl-*N*-nitrosothiazolidine, *Food and Chemical Toxicol.*, **22**(4), 253–9.

Voogd, C. E., van der Stel, J. J., and Jacobs, J. J. J. A. A. (1979). The mutagenic action of nitroimidazoles. IV. A comparison of the mutagenic action of several nitroimidazoles and some imidazoles, *Mutation Res.*, **66**(3), 207–21.

Wei, C. I., Kitamura, K., and Shibamoto, T. (1981). Mutagenicity of Maillard browning products obtained from a starch–glycine model system, *Food and Cosmetics Toxicol.*, **79**, 749–51.

Yamaguchi, T., and Nakagawa, K. (1983). Mutagenicity of and formation of oxygen radicals by trioses and glyoxal derivatives, *Agric. Biol. Chem.*, **47**(11), 2461–5.

Yamamoto, T., Tsuji, K., Kosuge, T., Okamoto, T., Shudo, K., Takeda, K., Iitake, Y., Yamaguchi, K., Seino, Y., Yahagi, T., Nagao, M., and Sugimura, T. (1978). Isolation and structure determination of mutagenic substances in L-glutamic acid pyrolysates, *Proc. Japan Academy*, **54B**, 248–50.

Yen, G. C., and Chau, C. F. (1993). Inhibition by xylose–lysine Maillard reaction products of the formation of MeIQx in a heated creatinine, glycine, and glucose model system, *Biosci., Biotechnol. Biochem.*, **57**(4), 664–5.

Yen, G. C., and Hsieh, P. P. (1994). Possible mechanisms of antimutagenic effect of Maillard reaction products prepared from xylose and lysine, *J. Agric. Food Chem.*, **42**, 133–7.

Yen, G. C., and Lee, T. C. (1986). Mutagen formation in the reaction of Maillard reaction products, 2-acetylpyrrole and its analogs with nitrite, *Food Chem. Toxicol.*, **24**(12), 1303–8.

Yen, G. C., Tsai, L. C., and Lii, J. D. (1992). Antimutagenic effect of Maillard browning products obtained from amino acids and sugars, *Food Chem. Toxicol.*, **30**(2), 127–2.

Yoshida, D., and Okamoto, H. (1980). Formation of mutagens by heating the aqueous solution of amino acids and some nitrogenous compounds with addition of glucose, *Agric. Biol. Chem.*, **44**, 2521–2.

Yoshida, D., Matsumoto, T., Okamoto, H., Mizusaki, S., Kushi, A., and Fukuhara, Y. (1986). Formation of mutagens by heating foods and model systems, *Environ. Health Perspect.*, **67**, 55–8.

Yoshida, D., Matsumoto, T., Yoshimura, R., and Matsuzaki, T. (1978). Mutagenicity of amino-α-carbolines in pyrolysis products of soybean globulin, *Biochem. Biophys. Commun.*, **83**, 915–20.

8

DNA-Advanced Glycosylation

RICHARD BUCALA and ANTHONY CERAMI

The Picower Institute for Medical Research, Manhasset, New York, USA

INTRODUCTION

The central role of DNA mutations in cancer has provided much impetus for identifying important mediators of DNA damage *in vivo*. Although numerous exogenous sources of DNA damage have been studied over the years, such as radiation and chemical mutagens, increasing evidence suggests that agents arising from 'endogenous' biochemical processes may play a particularly important role in producing DNA mutations and initiating oncogenic transformation. The majority of human cancers occur as a function of chronological age and the genomic DNA present within long-lived cells is susceptible to the slow accumulation of age-dependent forms of damage.[1-3] Among the age-associated changes in DNA that have been documented are an increased frequency of chromosomal aberrations and karyotype instability, and an increased level of nucleotide modification, DNA crosslinks and DNA strand-breaks.[4-11]

Over the last several years, we have been studying DNA-advanced glycosylation: the biochemical and genetic consequences that result from the interaction of reducing sugars with DNA nucleotides. We review studies indicating that not only is DNA susceptible to modification by reducing sugars, but that these modification reactions produce a unique spectrum of mutations which are manifested by DNA transposition. Recent investigations also have led to the structural identification of model, AGE nucleotides which should provide a future basis for measuring AGE-mediated DNA damage *in vivo*.

The Maillard Reaction: Consequences for the Chemical and Life Sciences. Edited by Raphael Ikan
©1996 John Wiley & Sons Ltd

ADVANCED GLYCOSYLATION:
THE MAILLARD REACTION *IN VIVO*

Although reactions between reducing sugars and amines were described first by Maillard over 80 years ago, it is only within the last 15–20 years that there has been an appreciation of the fact that similar chemical processes occur *in vivo*. These reactions have come to be termed 'advanced glycosylation', in part to distinguish the Maillard products that arise *in vivo* from those that form under the harsh, nonphysiological conditions that occur during the heating or storage of foodstuffs. By a variety of chemical criteria, it now has become apparent that 'early' nonenzymatic glycosylation products readily undergo additional inter- and intramolecular rearrangements *in vivo* to produce a heterogenous group of irreversibly bound, crosslinking moieties. Like Maillard products, these compounds, called advanced glycosylation end-products or AGEs, possess distinctive fluorescent and crosslinking properties. AGEs accumulate most noticeably on long-lived tissue macromolecules. Nevertheless, the precise chemical structures of the AGEs that form *in vivo* remain largely unknown.[12,13]

Figure 8.1 illustrates the structures of several AGE compounds that have been described and studied to date.[14–19] These products were purified from model glucose–protein incubations or isolated directly from aged connective tissue proteins. The compound FFI (furoyl-furanyl imidazole) was the first chemically defined AGE that was proposed to form in human tissues and exhibits the covalent, crosslinking potential of glucose-derived Amadori products.[14] Although subsequent mechanistic studies indicate that most of the FFI present in proteins forms by the incorporation of free NH_3, there is evidence to suggest that structures that are immunochemically similar to FFI do exist *in vivo*.[20–24] Pyrrole-containing compounds such as AFGP and pyrraline also have been isolated from model *in vitro* incubation mixtures;[15,17] however, it is unclear whether AGEs such as pyrraline in fact form on long-lived connective tissue proteins.[25,26] Pentosidine is a lysine–arginine crosslink which was purified from aged connective tissue collagen.[18] Although originally postulated to arise from pentoses, pentosidine was found to also form from the reaction of hexoses with proteins.[27,28] Sensitive HPLC methods for the detection of pentosidine have been devised and have confirmed its presence in aged and diabetic tissues.[29,30] Nevertheless, pentosidine was isolated on the basis of its acid stability and fluorescent properties and quantitative considerations suggest that pentosidine accounts for only a small percentage ($< 1.0\%$) of the glucose-derived crosslinks that form under *in vivo* conditions. Thus, the precise identity of the predominant AGE structures that occur *in vivo* remains unknown. Detailed immunochemical analyses, for example, have shown that a major class of cross-reactive AGE epitopes forms *in vivo* on diverse protein and lipid substrates.[31–33] These epitopes are acid labile and

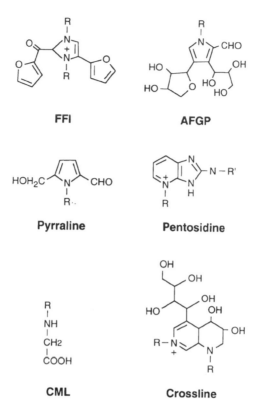

Figure 8.1. Structure of various chemically defined AGEs. R denotes the potential lysine and RR′ the arginine backbones respectively. (Modified from Ref. 12)

appear structurally distinct from any of the chemically defined AGEs that have been described thus far.

A large body of data has now established that AGEs alter the structural and functional properties of proteins, and many of these alterations have been linked to the pathophysiological changes that accompany both long-standing diabetes and normal aging. AGEs progressively crosslink tissue and arterial collagen and act to increase connective tissue rigidity.[34,35] This contributes to the vascular and ligamentous rigidity which accompanies normal aging and which is accelerated by diabetes mellitus. Protein-linked AGEs also act as reactive foci to covalently trap circulating serum proteins such as albumin, immunoglobulins and lipoproteins.[36,37] This may account in part for the increase in protein deposition and in basement membrane thickening that occurs in the systemic and renal vasculature of diabetic patients. Cell surface receptors that are specific for the recognition, uptake and degradation of AGE-modified proteins have been identified on circulating monocytes, endothelial

cells and renal mesangial cells.[38–41] AGEs are chemotactic for monocytes, and
the receptor-mediated uptake of AGE-modified proteins initiates cytokine-
mediated processes that can promote tissue remodeling or, under pathophysiological circumstances in the kidney, contribute to excessive matrix
production and glomerulosclerosis.[42–44] Occupancy of endothelial receptors
by AGEs leads to increased vascular permeability, down-regulation of the
anticoagulant factor thrombomodulin and increased synthesis of the proco-
agulant tissue factor.[44,45]

Recent studies also have suggested an important role *in vivo* for AGE-
mediated redox reactions. For instance, AGEs have been shown to chemically
inactivate the radical-based, endothelial-derived relaxing factor, nitric oxide.[46]
The progressive accumulation of AGEs on subendothelial collagen may thus
account for the impairment of endothelium-dependent, nitric oxide respon-
siveness which develops in diabetic and aged vasculature.[46,47] More recently,
redox active AGEs have been implicated in the initiation of fatty acid
oxidation.[33] Experimentally, these oxidative reactions occur independently of
any of the metal-catalyzed, free radical processes that have been hypothesized
in the past to be necessary for the formation of lipid oxidation products. The
formation of AGEs on low-density lipoprotein (LDL), which has been shown
to occur readily *in vivo*,[33,48] may explain the origin of oxidized-LDL, a
particularly atherogenic form of this lipoprotein. AGE modification of LDL
has also been shown to interfere with its normal uptake by tissue LDL
receptors, contributing in part to the dyslipidemia that occurs in patients with
diabetes or renal insufficiency.[48]

DNA-ADVANCED GLYCOSYLATION
IN PROKARYOTIC SYSTEMS

Several years ago we began an experimental program aimed at investigating the
possibility that DNA nucleotides might also react with reducing sugars to
initiate advanced glycosylation reactions. Although the position of primary
amino groups on the delocalized ring systems of nucleotide bases renders them
less nucleophilic than either the α or the ε amino groups of protein amino acids,
it was reasoned that the extremely long residence time of DNA molecules in
resting, nondividing cells might favor the gradual, time-dependent accumulation of DNA-linked AGEs. In model studies, it was observed that incubation
of individual nucleotides or purified DNA with reducing sugars at 37 °C
produced moieties with similar absorbance and fluorescence properties as the
products that form during the advanced glycosylation of proteins (Figure 8.2).
GMP–AGE products showed the highest fluorescence yield, followed by the
AMP- and the CMP-derived advanced glycosylation product(s). As expected,
spectral changes were not detected in the case of the nucleotide TMP, which

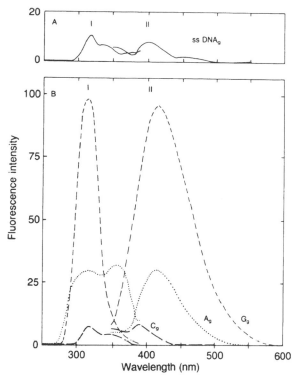

Figure 8.2. Excitation (I) and emission (II) difference spectra (uncorrected) for G6P-modified single-stranded DNA and nucleotides. Fluorescent intensity is expressed in arbitrary units. A: AGE-modified single-stranded DNA (ssDNA$_g$). B: G6P-modified AMP (A$_g$), CMP (C$_g$), and GMP (G$_g$). (Modified from Ref. 49)

lacks a primary amino group. Single-stranded DNA showed markedly greater absorbance and fluorescent changes than double-stranded DNA, presumably because intrastrand hydrogen bonding renders the amino groups of double-stranded DNA less accessible to interaction with reducing sugars.[49]

We next investigated the effect of advanced glycosylation on the biological activity of DNA from the single-stranded *Escherichia coli* bacteriophage f1. Purified DNA was incubated with reducing sugars (glucose or glucose-6-phosphate (G6P)) and then transfected into *E. coli* to measure viral plaque formation. Viral DNA that had been incubated with sugars showed a dramatic decrease in transfection efficiency: incubation with 150 mM G6P for 8 days decreased viral plaque formation by 4 orders of magnitude. Glucose, which has a diminished ability to glycosylate proteins relative to G6P, caused a smaller decrease in transfection efficiency: at 150 mM, transfection capacity was reduced to 33% of control.[49]

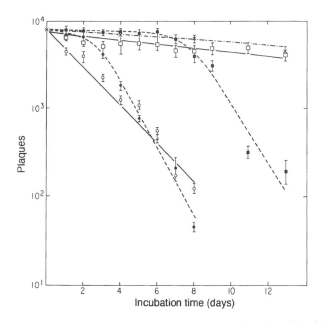

Figure 8.3. Rate of fl DNA inactivation by 25 mM G6P (○, 25 mM glucose (□), 25 mM G6P + 5 mM Boc-lysine (●) and 25 mM glucose + 5 mM Boc-lysine (■). Control DNA incubated with Boc-lysine alone (×). (Modified from Ref. 49)

Native fl DNA exists as a covalently closed circle. Gel electrophoresis analysis showed that G6P modification was associated with a time-dependent conversion of closed circular fl DNA into nicked, linear forms. Subsequent fluorographic analyses of incubations which contained $[^{14}C]$-G6P demonstrated the incorporation of radiolabeled carbon into both closed-circular and linear DNA forms, indicating that the formation of a G6P–nucleotide adduct precedes DNA strand scission. Taken together, these data were consistent with the concept that reducing sugars covalently modify the primary amino groups of DNA, leading first to labilization of the nucleotide–deoxyribose glycosidic bone, then to β-elimination and phosphodiester bond cleavage.[49]

Follow-up studies revealed that the loss of transfection efficiency of glucose- or G6P-modified fl DNA could be markedly potentiated by the simultaneous inclusion of lysine in the incubation mixtures (Figure 8.3). Furthermore, radiolabeled lysine was observed to form covalent, acid-stable complexes with the DNA polynucleotide backbone. These data led to the concept that early, non-enzymatic glycoslation products produce an 'AGE-reactive intermediate' which then reacts with DNA more rapidly than glucose itself.[50]

The specific, DNA-damaging effects of reducing sugars and sugar/lysine co-

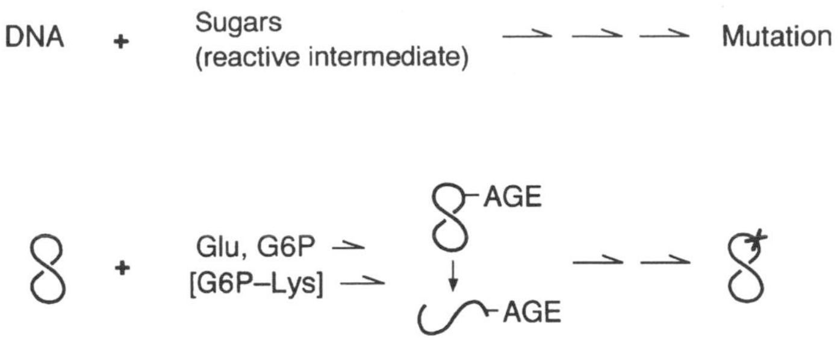

Figure 8.4. Generalized scheme for the interaction of reducing sugars with closed-circular plasmid DNA

incubation reactions naturally prompted investigation into the mutagenicity of AGE-modified DNA. In bacterial transformation studies, the plasmid pBR322 was modified by advanced glycosylation *in vitro* and screened for the loss of function of one of its two antibiotic resistance genes. AGE-modified DNA thus was observed to be mutagenized in a concentration- and time-dependent fashion.[51] In these experiments, the mutagenic activity of glucose–DNA incubations could also be greatly enhanced by the pre-incubation of glucose with lysine prior to addition to plasmid DNA. Figure 8.4 illustrates an overall scheme for the interaction of reducing sugars with plasmid DNA, leading to adduct formation, strand scission and mutation.

To investigate the direct mutagenic activity of reducing sugars *in vivo*, Lee and Cerami studied plasmid mutations in *E. coli* strains which were defective in the glycolytic enzymes phosphoglucose isomerase (strain DF40) or both phosphoglucose isomerase and glucose-6-phosphatase (strain DF2000).[52] These mutant strains grow well in the presence of gluconate as a carbon source but accumulate G6P intracellularly when glucose is added to the medium. In this experimental system, the mutation frequency of a plasmid-encoded marker gene, β-galactosidase, was assayed 24 hours after transfection and replication in an *E. coli* host which had either normal or elevated intracellular G6P levels. When compared to control conditions, seven- and thirteenfold increases in plasmid-encoded β-galactosidase mutations were observed in the strains DF40 and DF2000 when the intracellular G6P levels were increased twenty- and thirtyfold, respectively.[52]

It soon became evident that AGE-mediated mutations were associated with an unusual spectrum of structural changes in the target genes. In the case of mutant plasmids which were isolated after transfection into *E. coli* hosts, restriction enzyme mapping revealed that in many cases the affected plasmid genes had undergone gross DNA alterations, including insertions and deletions of large ($\geqslant 50$ bp) DNA fragments. What was even more intriguing was that the inserted DNA fragments could be identified by Southern hybridization to have arisen from host-derived DNA sequences.[51] Transposition of host DNA occurred in plasmids that had been modified by advanced glycosylation *in vitro*, as well as in native plasmids carried by the *E. coli* strains which accumulated high intracellular levels of G6P. These DNA insertions were identified subsequently to comprise sequences derived from known *E. coli* transposable elements such as INS-1 and $\gamma\delta$.[51,53] These transposable elements generally reside stably integrated within the bacterial host genome and can be associated with genes conferring antibiotic resistance to the host. Bacterial transpositions also possess terminal repeats which serve as recognition sequences for DNA integration, and certain elements may themselves code for 'transposase' enzymes which act to transfer the element from one site of integration to another. The induction of DNA transpositions by DNA–AGEs was completely unanticipated, given the initial concept that AGE modification leads to the formation of bulky, nucleotide adducts that might in turn be substrates for simple, excisional repair systems. Rather, it was apparent that AGE-induced DNA damage serves as an important inducing signal for DNA transposition. In separate experiments, it was also observed that the presence within the bacterial chromosome of another transposable element, Tn5 or Tn10, increased markedly the rate of $\gamma\delta$ movement into AGE-modified plasmids.[53]

In summary, it was demonstrated that DNA–AGEs form readily *in vivo* in short-lived prokaryotic cells and that AGE modification produces mutations in part as the result of a novel, DNA-transpositional activity. There have been extremely few agents or signals that have been identified to elicit DNA transposition in bacteria and the possibility that AGE-mediated signals subserve this function has important implications both for the physiology and the evolution of prokaryotic genomes.

DNA-ADVANCED GLYCOSYLATION IN EUKARYOTIC SYSTEMS

The induction of DNA transposition by AGEs in bacteria then prompted a search for a similar inducible activity in higher, eukaryotic cells. Until recently, evidence for the existence of transposable elements in mammalian genomes has been largely indirect and has been based on certain structural features shared by widely dispersed repetitive DNA families, such as the SINEs (short-interspersed repetitive elements such as *Alu*) and LINEs (long-interspersed repetitive elements).[54,55] Within the last several years, *Alu*-containing insertions have been found to mutate a number of human genes, including those for the LDL receptor, the *Miv* oncogene, ornithine δ-aminotransferase, cholinesterase and the neurofibromatosis NF1 gene.[56–60] Recent studies of the L1 repetitive elements have also identified a gene for reverse transcriptase that may mediate certain retro-transposition events in eukaryotic cells.[61]

To investigate the role of advanced glycosylation in the transposition of mammalian DNA, we studied the effect of AGE modification on a 'shuttle vector' plasmid (pPy35) containing the *lacI* gene as a mutagenesis marker. Shuttle vectors contain both a prokaryotic and a eukaryotic origin of replication, thus permitting them to be passaged first in mammalian cells and then transferred to bacteria for amplification and large-scale mutational screening. The pPy35 plasmid thus contains both the mouse polyoma virus and the pBR322 origins of replication. Also present are the genes for neomycin and ampicillin resistance which permits selectable growth in eukaryotic and prokaryotic cells respectively. Purified, shuttle vector DNA (pPy35) was modified by advanced glycosylation *in vitro* and transfected into the murine lymphoid cell line X63Ag8.653. After selection in neomycin-supplemented tissue culture medium, the murine cells were harvested and the episomal DNA purified and assayed for *lacI* mutations by α-complementation in the *E. coli* host MC1061. The mutation rate for *lacI* was found to increase from 0.1% for control, unmodified plasmids to as high as 28% for AGE-modified plasmids.[62] Overall, these results were consistent with those observed previously for AGE mutagenesis in bacteria.

Shuttle vector DNA then was isolated and analyzed for size differences by gel electrophoresis and restriction enzyme analysis. The majority of plasmid mutations were found to be associated with large ($\geqslant 100\,bp$) net insertion or deletion of DNA. Of interest, the mutant population obtained after DNA modification showed an apparent increase in the proportion of plasmids with DNA insertions and a corresponding decrease in the proportion of plasmids with DNA deletions or without a net DNA size change. Restriction enzyme mapping revealed that each DNA insertion disrupted the plasmid *lacI* gene and Southern hybridization confirmed that the DNA insertions were homologous to sequences present in mouse genomic DNA.[62]

Three DNA insertions, designated INS-1 (0.8 kB), INS-2 (1.5 kB) and INS-3 (4 kB), were identified by partial sequence analysis and chosen for further study. Oligonucleotide primers specific for unique, sequenced regions of the INS-1, INS-2 and INS-3 insertions were then used in polymerase chain reactions to screen for related elements in 92 insertion-containing mutant plasmids chosen from 15 independent transfection experiments. The INS-1-specific primers were found to amplify a common DNA sequence in 13 of the insertion-containing plasmids isolated from 9 independent transfections. Mutant plasmids isolated from control (non-AGE modified) DNA transfections also contained examples of the INS-1 element, albeit at a much lower frequency. The identity of the INS-1 element in multiple, independent transfections was then confirmed by DNA sequencing of the INS-1 insertion

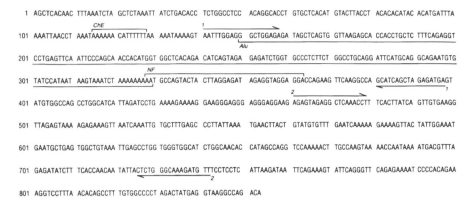

Figure 8.5. DNA sequence of the eukaryotic insertion element INS-1. The two sets of amplification primers used to screen insertion-containing mutants are indicated ('1', '2'). Also shown are the 179 bp region with homology (78%) to the murine B1 repetitive element or *Alu* homolog ('Alu'), the sequence common to the two direct repeats present at the ends of a 342 bp *Alu* insertion identified in the cholinesterase gene of a family afflicted with acholinesterasemia ('ChE') and a 36 bp region with 75% homology to an *Alu*-containing insertion described in a patient with neurofibromatosis ('NF'). (Modified from Ref. 62)

in four clones, each isolated from an independent transfection. The incidence of total plasmid mutations attributed to transposition of the INS-1 element was calculated to increase sixtyfold after AGE modification (0.025 to 1.4–1.6%).[62]

The complete DNA sequence and notable features of the 853 bp INS-1 element are shown in Figure 8.5. The INS-1 element contains a 179 bp region bearing 78% homology to the B1 repetitive sequence superfamily, the murine equivalent of the human *Alu* sequence. Of interest, regions of homology were also found between INS-1 and two recently described insertion sequences causing mutations in human genes. Within INS-1 is one of the two direct repeats (AAAAAAXATTTTTT) that flank a 342 base pair *Alu*-type insertion found to disrupt the cholinesterase gene in a Japanese family afflicted with acholinesterasemia.[59] Also present is a short (36 bp) region outside the B1 element that is partially homologous (75%) to an *Alu*-containing insertion identified in a patient with neurofibromatosis.[60] The four sequenced examples of complete INS-1 elements were found to be located within a 392–683 bp size deletion in *lacl* that varied in position between nucleotides 309 and 992 of the *lac* sequence. Examination of the INS-1 sequence and the plasmid *lacl* flanking regions revealed no apparent sequence homologies or repetitive regions.[62]

Additional DNA sequencing analyses of the INS-2 and INS-3 elements revealed the presence of an INS-1 partial sequence comprising nucleotides 329–853 (Figure 8.6). Apparent truncation of the INS-1 sequence occurred

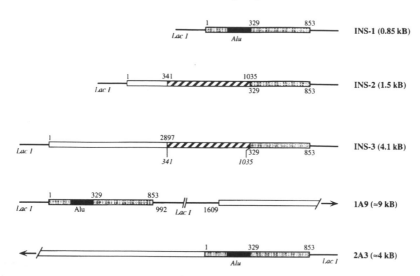

Figure 8.6. Summary of insertion sequences isolated from AGE-modified plasmid clones. The INS-1 element shown is representative of four insertional mutants isolated from independent transfections. Identical regions are indicated by similar shading and unique sequence is represented by the open, unshaded segments. *Lac* sequencee is indicated by the solid line. Also shown are the partially determined structures of the large 1A9 and 2A3 *lacl*⁻ clones. (Modified from Ref. 62)

immediately 3' to the *Alu* homologous segment. Figure 8.6 also shows the partial structures of two additional *lacl* clones, designated 1A9 and 2A3. The 1A9 clone was found to contain two insertions, a complete INS-1 and an ≈8 kB element separated by 700 bp of intervening *lacl* sequence. The large 2A3 clone contained an INS-1 element linked at its 5' end with ≈4 kB of an additional DNA insertion.

A role for *Alu* DNA in eukaryotic transposition was originally suggested by structural homology with the highly conserved 7SL RNA sequence and by the widespread genomic dispersion of *Alu* sequences.[54,55] Recent studies also have revealed specific examples of gene disruption by *Alu* DNA.[56–60] The molecular mechanisms responsible for the transposition of the *Alu*-containing INS-1 element remain to be elucidated. Neither flanking repeats nor an open reading frame that might code for a transposase-like enzyme were found within the INS-1 insertion. The fact that all of the sequenced examples of INS-1 were present as a DNA insertion superimposed over a deletion suggests that DNA recombination may be a necessary feature of INS-1 integration. This is supported by the appearance of clones in which the INS-1 sequence is flanked by additional host-derived sequences, and by examples of apparent truncation of the INS-1 element immediately 3' to the region of *Alu* homology (Figure 8.6).

In more recent experiments, we utilized AGE-modified shuttle vector DNA to investigate INS-1 insertional mutagenesis in additional cell types. Mutations resulting from the insertion of INS-1 elements were identified by transfecting AGE-modified plasmids into the mouse T-cell line ASL-1, the human monocyte line THP-1 and the human T-cell line Jurkat. Southern hybridization analysis using murine INS-1 as a probe revealed an INS-1 insertional frequency of 0.26% for mouse ASL-1 cells and 0.35% for human Jurkat cells. Control experiments performed in the absence of the AGE modification showed an INS-1 mutagenesis frequency which was <0.025% for both cell types. Thus, it is apparent that INS-1 transposition in response to AGE-modified DNA is neither a cell nor a species-specific phenomenon (unpublished observations).

In preliminary studies, INS-1 DNA probes have been used in Southern hybridizations with mouse genomic DNA to begin to assess the relative copy number and configuration of genomic INS-1 sequences. As expected for a repetitive sequence, DNA probes from the *Alu*-homologous region were found to hybridize to extensive, overlapping regions of restriction enzyme digestion patterns of mouse genomic DNA. In contrast, DNA probes derived from unique sequence regions of INS-1 showed hybridization to only two bands, suggesting that this sequence occurs infrequently and in relatively few copies in normal mouse DNA (unpublished observations).

Although the INS-1 sequence family does not appear to display any of the structural features that have been proposed to be characteristic of mobile, transposable elements (i.e. terminal repeats or transposase-encoding genes), they may nevertheless represent elements that are sensitive to the transposition-inducing or recombinogenic activities of AGE-modified DNA.

STRUCTURAL STUDIES OF DNA-ADVANCED GLYCOSYLATION END-PRODUCTS

Structural elucidation of AGEs that form *in vivo* remains a challenging problem. As noted earlier, AGEs form slowly, are chemically heterogeneous and generally can be isolated only in low yield. AGEs also tend to be labile to acid and base hydrolysis, making the isolation of products that are stably attached to macromolecules *in vivo* extremely difficult. Despite the fact that several protein-derived AGE products have been isolated over the years from either model *in vitro* reactions or from connective tissue specimens, the precise structures of the major protein-linked AGEs that occur *in vivo* remain largely undefined.

To approach the identification of AGE moieties on DNA, we recently embarked on the systematic examination of reaction products that form during the incubation of nucleotides with glucose and glucose-derived products. 'Fast' refluxing reactions were studied first so as to identify any potential products

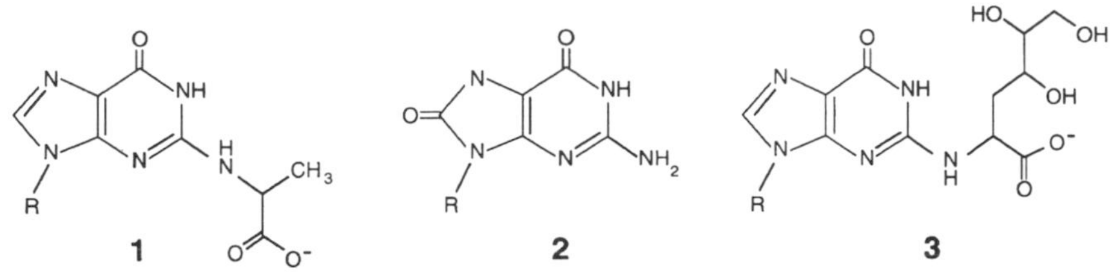

Figure 8.7. Structures of AGE-modified nucleotides or nucleotide bases

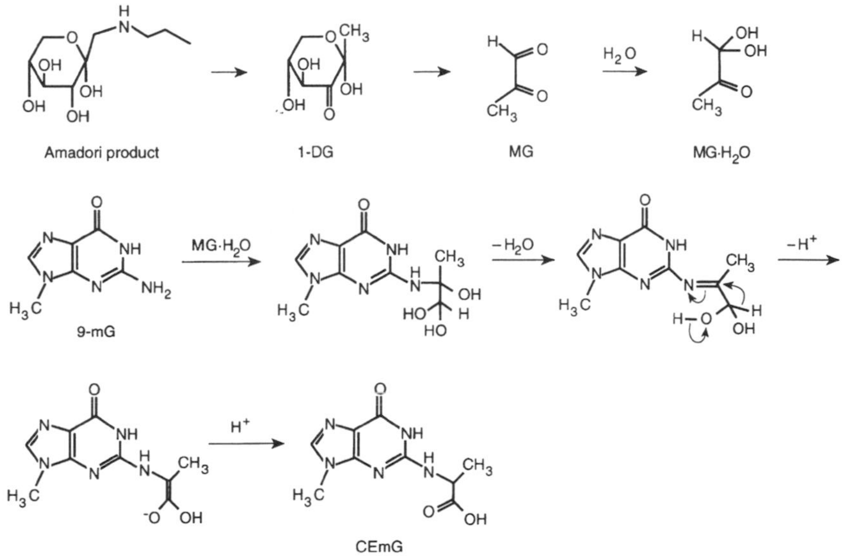

Figure 8.8. Proposed reaction pathway for the formation of the nucleotide–AGE: carboxyethylguanine, MG: methylglyoxal, CEmG: N^2-(1-carboxyethyl)-9-methylguanine. (Modified from Ref. 64)

that might form in high yield. The presence of candidate nucleotide–AGEs were then searched for in 'long-term' incubations performed at 37 °C. The glucose-derived reactants used in these incubations included 1-n-propylamino-*N*-D-glucoside (a Schiff base), 1-n-propylamino-D-fructose (an Amadori product) and 3-deoxyglucosone (3-DG), a previously identified, reactive Amadori breakdown product.[63] All incubations were performed with nucleotides bearing a methyl substituent in place of the naturally occurring deoxyribose structure. This served to preserve the natural electronic configuration and reactivity of amino groups in the nucleotide base. At the same time, the methyl proton resonances were useful diagnostic tools, indicating the number and approximate abundances of different products in crude reaction mixtures.

9-Methyladenine was not observed to react to any observable extent with glucose or any of the glucose-derived reactants. 1-Methylcytosine was somewhat reactive towards G6P and G6P/Lys and trace amounts of products were detected by ^{1}H-NMR after two days of reflux. 9-Methylguanine showed the highest reactivity in these studies. It reacted with D-glucose, G6P, G6P/Lys and the glucose-derived Schiff base and Amadori product. In all reactions, the major product was identified by NMR and mass spectroscopy to be a guanine substituted at the N^{-2} position by a 3-carbon carboxyethl moiety (Figure 8.7, **1**). The structure of the isolated nucleotide (N^2-1(1-carboxyethyl)guanine, or CEG) was independently confirmed by the reaction of 9-methylguanine with methylglyoxal (MG). Methylglyoxal is a known Maillard product which can form by retro-aldol fission of 1-deoxyglucosone (1-DG), an Amadori decomposition product.[63] A proposed scheme for the formation of CEG from 9-methylguanine and Amadori product is shown in Figure 8.8. Methylglyoxal is positive in the Ames test and transfection studies showed that methylgloxal-modified plasmid DNA is also mutagenized in eukaryotic cells.[64]

A second base, 8-oxo-7-H-9-methylguanine (OmG), was additionally identified to form in long-term reactions of 9-methylguanine and glucose (Figure 8.7, **2**). The OmG tautomer, 8-hydroxyguanine, was originally described to be produced in DNA exposed to ionizing radiation or to radical-generating agents.[65] Hydroxylation of guanine at the C-8 position has also been reported to occur when 2-deoxyguanosine or DNA is heated with solid glucose.[66] 8-Hydroxyguanine has been reported to be present in appreciable amounts in human urine, and its concentration may reflect host age or basal metabolic rate. Ames and coworkers have suggested that the presence of this base may indicate the cumulative exposure of DNA to reactive oxygen species.[67] Although reducing sugars have been shown to produce oxygen free radicals by metal-catalyzed autoxidation *in vitro*, significant autoxidation is unlikely to occur *in vivo*. It is possible, therefore, that OmG may also arise *in vivo* from strictly glucose-dependent, Maillard processes. This question may be addressed, for example, by examining OmG/8-hydroxyguanine levels in diabetic tissues, where the content of Maillard products is increased markedly.

Knerr and coworkers have reported the occurrence of nucleotide glycation products isolated from the incubation of glucose, guanosine and propylamine at 37 °C in concentrated phosphate buffer.[68,69] In addition to an N^2-glycosylated guanine, an N^2-substituted trihydroxyhexanaoic acid was identified to be present (Figure 8.7, **3**). This product appears to form from the reaction of guanosine with 3-DG, another well-described Amadori product degradation product.

It is important to note that many products arising from amine-catalyzed advanced glycosylation reactions *in vivo* are chemically analogous to the Maillard products that arise during the heating and storage of foodstuffs.

Many of the compounds that form during these *ex vivo* sugar–amine condensation reactions have been identified to exhibit DNA-breaking, mutagenic and tumor-promoting activity in different experimental test systems.[70-72] Maillard reaction products, for instance, have been shown to induce chromosomal aberrations in Chinese hamster ovary cells and to initiate gene conversion in the yeast *Saccharomyces cerevisiae*.[73,74] Among the compounds present in cooked foods that have been implicated in these genotoxic effects are the heterocyclic amines imidazoquinoline and imidazoquinoxaline (collectively termed 'IQ' compounds).[75] Alternatively, other Maillard reaction products have been shown to protect against the mutagenic activity compounds such as nitrosoamines.[76]

BIOLOGICAL CONSEQUENCES OF DNA-ADVANCED GLYCOSYLATION

In addition to the damaging effects of advanced glycosylation on genomic DNA, numerous other potentially important sources of DNA damage have been described over the years. Intrinsic oxidants, for example, are produced by cellular metabolism, particularly by those enzymatic pathways that reduce molecular oxygen and generate oxygen free radicals at a low, basal rate. It has been estimated that oxidative damage produces hundreds of modified DNA residues per cell per day, and accounts for the 8-hydroxyguanine, thymine glycol and other nucleotide derivatives that are readily detected in urine.[77,78] Additional extrinsic sources of oxidative damage include the radiolytic reactions initiated by background levels of γ- and X-ray radiation. Energy from these radiations produces free radicals that can react directly with nucleotide bases.[79] These lesions have been hypothesized to provide a steady source of nucleotide misincorporation and DNA mutations that contribute potentially to 'error catastrophe' and cellular senescence.[80,81]

The age-dependent accumulation of AGE products in mammalian tissues and the presence of specific scavenger receptor systems that internalize AGEs suggest that there is continual intracellular exposure to reactive AGE products. Nevertheless, kinetic considerations suggest that AGE-mediated DNA damage is likely to occur at a lower frequency than either oxidation or thermally induced depurination events, which have been estimated to affect 10 000 nucleotides per cell per day.[49,82] Depurination also leads slowly to phosphodiester bond hydrolysis and DNA strand-breakage.[83] Although some studies indicate that DNA strand-breakage increases with age, other investigations have failed to confirm this finding, suggesting that efficient mechanisms exist to repair these lesions.[84,85] The mutagenic potential of various forms of DNA damage thus varies directly with the capacity of cells to enzymatically repair particular nucleotide adducts. Therefore, the precise contribution of DNA-advanced glycosylation reactions to the cumulative effect of various sources of DNA damage is difficult to assess at the present time. Nevertheless, the high estimated frequencies attributed to certain processes such as spontaneous or thermally induced depurination *in vitro* suggest that DNA repair mechanisms function efficiently to prevent most of these forms of mutagenic injury.[86,87] Because an important biological effect of AGE formation on proteins is crosslink formation, intranuclear-advanced glycosylation reactions could readily account for the increase in DNA–protein and DNA–DNA crosslinking that has been observed to occur in aged tissue.[10] If AGE-mediated DNA damage in fact leads to the formation of covalent crosslinks, the limited capacity of cells to repair DNA crosslinks indicates that DNA-advanced glycosylation may be a particularly dangerous source of 'intrinsic' age-dependent damage.[88] It may be impossible for cells to escape this form of lethal damage other than by drastic recombination or transposition events.

Numerous studies over the years which have relied on cytogenetic techniques or the selection of mutated loci *in vitro* have led to the concept that genomic mutations increase with age. DNA–AGEs may play an important role in the increased frequency of chromosomal abnormalities (translocations, deletions, etc.) that occur during aging. Chromosomal rearrangements were among the first DNA abnormalities described to be associated with normal aging.[82,89–91] In addition, there appears to be a close association between karyotype (chromosome) abnormalities and cancer, the prevalence of which increases markedly with age.[90,91] In tumor types that have been associated with specific karyotype abnormalities, chromosomal rearrangements have been shown in several instances to either activate a cellular oncogene or to inactivate a tumor suppressor gene.[91,92] It has recently been noted that chromosomal transloca-tions at the locus associated with B-cell leukemia/lymphoma-2 (BCL2), for example, occurs more commonly in the B cells of aged individuals than in younger individuals.[92] The acquisition and accumulation of chromosomal aberrations ultimately may underlie the age-dependent incidence of several tumors, including various leukemias/lymphomas, colon, lung and breast carcinomas, and brain tumors.[1–3,93,94]

Within the context of aging, a time-dependent decline in the functional capacity of cells to repair DNA damage has been invoked as an important mechanism for cellular aging.[1,86,87] Although there have been some data to support a role for DNA repair pathways in species longevity, many investigations have failed to find either consistent or significantly different levels of DNA repair capacity in young versus aged cells or tissues.[95,96] The proposition that DNA mutations increase with age has been affirmed recently *in vivo* in a transgenic mouse model of aging. In this study, it was observed that spontaneous mutations in a nonselectable transgene, *lacI*, increased approxi-mately fourfold over a two year age span.[97]

Our own biological studies have focused more closely on the role of DNA-advanced glycosylation in the teratogenic effect of maternal hyperglycemia.[98] Congenital malformations affecting multiple organ systems are responsible for approximately 50% of the perinatal deaths in infants of insulin-dependent diabetic mothers and, among surviving infants, birth defects are at least 3 times more frequent than in those born to nondiabetic mothers.[99,100] Maternal glucose passes freely through the placenta and fetal serum glucose levels have been shown to reflect closely the levels present in the mother. To address the possibility that maternal hyperglycemia contributes to mutagenesis in fetal DNA, we studied mouse embryos that were transgenic for the *lacI* mutagenesis reporter gene. Three to four day old blastocysts were transferred into the uterine horns of pseudopregnant female mice which were previously rendered diabetic by streptozotocin treatment. The embryos were allowed to develop and the genomic DNA then assayed for the occurrence of *lacI* mutations. Embryo transfer was necessary to eliminate any potential mutagenic effects of streptozotocin, the agent used to induce diabetes in the host mice. These experiments showed that despite the short (21 day) gestational period of the mouse, a statistically significant twofold increase in the mutant frequency of the *lacI* transgene occurred in fetuses that developed in a mild diabetic environment compared to those that developed under normoglycemic conditions. Although it remains to be established that these mutations were due directly to the effect of DNA-advanced glycosylation, these data provide important evidence for the mutagenicity of a cellular environment high in glucose and AGEs.[98]

CONCLUSION

Increasing evidence over the years has established that AGE products do indeed form in mammalian tissues. The possibility that DNA-advanced glycosylation reactions occur *in vivo* provides an important unifying concept for understanding the role of biochemical aging processes in the etiology of age-associated karyotype instability and chromosomal aberrations leading to cancer. Future studies aimed at detecting the prevalence of AGE–DNA products *in vivo* along with investigations into the mechanistic basis of AGE-mediated DNA transposition events should prove to be fruitful avenues of inquiry.

ACKNOWLEDGEMENTS

These studies were supported by NIH grant DK19655-15 and the Brookdale Foundation.

REFERENCES

1. C. E. Finch, *Longevity, Senescence and the Genome*, The University of Chicago Press, Chicago, 1990.
2. J. Brugge, T. Curran, E. Harlow and F. McCormick (eds.), *Origins of Human Cancer: A Comprehensive Review*, Cold Spring Harbor Laboratory Press, Cold Spring Harbor, New York, 1991.
3. J. Cairns, *Nature*, **289**, 353 (1981).
4. G. M. Martin, A. C. Smith, D. J. Ketterer, C. E. Ogburn and C. M. Disteche, *Israel J. Med. Sci.*, **21**, 296 (1985).
5. T. Lindahl, *Nature*, **362**, 709 (1993).
6. E. L. Schneider, in *Cytogenetics of Aging* (ed. E. L. Schneider), Plenum Press, New York, 1978.
7. C. B. Harley, A. B. Futcher, and C. W. Greider, *Nature*, **345**, 458 (1990).
8. E. Mullaart, P. H. M. Lohman, F. Berends and J. Vijg, *Mut. Res.*, **237**, 189 (1990).
9. K. Randerath, M. V. Reddy, and R. M. Disher. *Carcinogenesis*, 7, 1615 (1986).
10. J. J. Bojanovic, A. D. Jevtovic, V. S. Pantic, S. M. Dugandzic and D. S. Javonovic, *Gerontologia*, **16**, 304 (1970).
11. P. Crine and W. G. Verly, *Biochim. Biophys. Acta*, **442**, 50 (1976).
12. R. Bucala and A. Cerami, *Adv. Pharmacol.*, **23**, 1 (1992).
13. F. G. Njoroge and V. M. Monnier, in *The Maillard Reaction in Aging, Diabetes and Nutrition* (eds. J. W. Baynes and V. M. Monnier), Alan R. Liss, New York, 1989.
14. S. Pongor, P. C. Ulrich, F. A. Bencsath and A. Cerami, *Proc. Natl Acad. Sci. (USA)*, **81**, 2684 (1984).
15. J. Farmar, P. Ulrich and A. Cerami, *J. Org. Chem.*, **53**, 2346 (1988).
16. M. U. Ahmed, S. R. Thorpe and J. W. Baynes, *J. Biol. Chem.*, **261**, 4889 (1986).
17. F. G. Njoroge, L. M. Sayre and V. M. Monnier, *Carbohydrate Res.*, **167**, 211 (1987).
18. D. R. Sell and V. M. Monnier, *J. Biol. Chem.*, **264**, 21597 (1989).
19. K. Nakamura, T. Hasegawa, Y. Fukunaga and K. Ienaga, *J. Chem. Soc. Chem. Commun.*, **14**, 992 (1992).
20. F. G. Njoroge, A. A. Fernandes and V. M. Monnier, *J. Biol. Chem.*, **263**, 10646 (1988).
21. S. Horiuchi, M. Shiga, N. Araki, K. Takata, M. Saitoh and Y. Morino, *J. Biol. Chem.*, **263**, 18821 (1988).
22. J. C. F. Chang, P. C. Ulrich, R. Bucala and A. Cerami, *J. Biol. Chem.*, **260**, 7970 (1985).
23. T. Poli, A. Lapolla, B. Pelli, A. Sturaro, P. Traldi, G. Crepaldi and D. Fedele, *J. Diabetic Complications*, **2**, 25 (1988).
24. A. Lapolla, C. Gerhardinger, B. Pelli, A. Sturaro, E. Del Favero, P. Traldi, G. Crepaldi and D. Fedele, *Diabetes*, **39**, 57 (1990).
25. S. Miyata and V. M. Monnier, *J. Clin. Invest.*, **89**, 1102 (1992).
26. P. R. Smith, H. H. Somani, P. J. Thornalley, J. Benn and P. H. Sonksen, *Clin. Sci.*, **84**, 87 (1993).
27. S. Grandhee and V. M. Monnier, *J. Biol. Chem.*, **266**, 11649 (1991).
28. D. G. Dyer, J. A. Blackledge, S. R. Thorpe and J. W. Baynes, *J. Biol. Chem.*, **266**, 11654 (1991).
29. D. R. Sell and V. M. Monnier, *J. Clin. Invest.*, **85**, 380 (1990).
30. D. R. Sell, A. Lapolla, P. Odetti, J. Fogarty and V. M. Monnier, *Diabetes*, **41**, 1286 (1992).
31. Z. Makita, H. Vlassara, A. Cerami and R. Bucala, *J. Biol. Chem.*, **267**, 5133 (1992).

32. S. Horiuchi, N. Araki and Y. Morino, *J. Biol. Chem.*, **266**, 7329 (1991).
33. R. Bucala, Z. Makita, T. Koschinsky, A. Cerami and H. Vlassara, *Proc. Natl Acad. Sci. (USA)*, **90**, 6434 (1993).
34. V. M. Monnier, R. R. Kohn and A. Cerami, *Proc. Natl Acad. Sci. (USA)*, **81**, 583 (1984).
35. R. R. Kohn, A. Cerami and V. M. Monnier, *Diabetes*, **33**, 57 (1984).
36. M. Brownlee, S. Pongor and A. Cerami, *J. Exp. Med.*, **158**, 1739 (1983).
37. M. Brownlee, H. Vlassara and A. Cerami, *Diabetes*, **34**, 938 (1985).
38. H. Vlassara, M. Brownlee and A. Cerami, *Proc. Natl Acad. Sci. (USA)*, **82**, 5588 (1985).
39. Z. Yang, Z. Makita, Y. Horii, S. Brunelle, A. Cerami, P. Sehajpal, M. Suthanthiran and H. Vlassara, *J. Exp. Med.*, **174**, 515 (1991).
40. E. Y. Skolnick, Z. Yang, Z. Makita, S. Radoff, M. Kirstein and H. Vlassara, *J. Exp. Med.*, **174**, 931 (1991).
41. M. Neeper, A. M. Schmidt, J. Brett, S. D. Yan, F. Wang, Y. C. Pan, K. Elliston, D. Stern and A. Shaw, *J. Biol. Chem.*, **267**, 14998 (1992).
42. H. Vlassara, M. Brownlee, K. Manogue, C. Dinarello and A. Cerami, *Science*, **240**, 1546 (1988).
43. T. Doi, H. Vlassara, M. Kirstein, Y. Yamada, G. E. Striker and L. J. Striker, *Proc. Natl Acad. Sci. (USA)*, **89**, 2873 (1992).
44. C. Eposito, D. Stern, H. Gerlach and H. Vlassara, *J. Exp. Med.*, **170**, 1387 (1989).
45. M. Kirstein, J. Brett, S. Radoff, D. Stern and H. Vlassara, *Proc. Natl Acad. Sci. (USA)*, **87**, 9010 (1990).
46. R. Bucala, K. Tracey and A. Cerami, *J. Clin. Invest.*, **87**, 432 (1991).
47. M. Hogan, A. Cerami and R. Bucala, *J. Clin. Invest.*, **90**, 1110 (1992).
48. R. Bucala, Z. Makita, G. Vega, S. Grundy, T. Koschinsky, A. Cerami and H. Vlassara, *Proc. Natl Aad. Sci. (USA)*, **91**, 9441 (1994).
49. R. Bucala, P. Model and A. Cerami, *Proc. Natl Acad. Sci. (USA)*, **81**, 105 (1984).
50. A. T. Lee and A. Cerami, *Mut. Res.*, **179**, 151 (1987).
51. R. Bucala, P. Model, M. Russel and A. Cerami, *Proc. Natl Acad. Sci. (USA)*, **82**, 8439 (1985).
52. A. T. Lee and A. Cerami, *Proc. Natl Acad. Sci. (USA)*, **84**, 8311 (1987).
53. A. T. Lee and A. Cerami, *Mutation Res.*, **249**, 125 (1991).
54. P. Jagadeeswaran, B. G. Forget and S. M. Weissman, *Cell*, **26**, 141 (1981).
55. P. L. Deininger, in *Mobile DNA* (eds. D. E. Berg and M. M. Howe), American Society of Microbiology, Washington, 1989.
56. M. A. Lehrman, J. L. Goldstein, D. W. Russell and M. S. Brown, *Cell*, **48**, 827 (1987).
57. A. Economou-Pachnis and P. N. Tsichlis, *Nuc. Acids Res.*, **13**, 8379 (1985).
58. G. A. Mitchell, D. Labuda, G. Fontaine, J. M. Saudubray, J. P. Bonnefont, S. Lyonnet, L. C. Brody, G. Steel, C. Obie and D. Valle, *Proc. Natl Acad. Sci. (USA)*, **88**, 815 (1991).
59. K. Muratani, T. Hada, Y. Yamamoto, T. Kaneko, K. Shigeto, T. Ohue, J. Furuyama and K. Higashino, *Proc. Natl Acad. Sci. (USA)*, **88**, 11315 (1991).
60. M. Wallace, L. B. Andersen, A. M. Saulino, P. E. Gregory, T. W. Glover ad F. S. Collins, *Nature*, **353**, 864 (1991).
61. S. L. Mathias, A. F. Scott, H. H. Kazazian, J. D. Boeke and A. Gabriel, *Science*, **254**, 1808 (1991).
62. R. Buccala, A. T. Lee, L. Rourke and A. Cerami, *Proc. Natl Acad. Sci. (USA)*, **90**, 2666 (1993).
63. J. E. Hodge, *J. Agric. Food Chem.*, **1**, 928 (1953).

64. A. Papoulis, Y. Al-Abed and R. Bucala, *Biochemistry* (in press).
65. H. Kasai, H. Tanooka and S. Nishimura, *Gann*, **75**, 1037 (1984).
66. H. Kasai and S. Nishimura, *Environmental Health Perspectives*, **67**, 111 (1986).
67. C. G. Fraga, M. K. Shigenaga, J. W. Park, P. Degan and B. N. Ames, *Proc. Natl Acad. Sci. (USA)*, **87**, 4533 (1990).
68. T. Knerr, S. Ochs and T. Severin, *Carbohydrate Res.*, **256**, 177 (1994).
69. T. Knerr and T. Severin, *Tetrahedron Lett.*, **34**, 7389 (1994).
70. K. Hiramoto, K. Kido and K. Kikugawa, *J. Agric. Food Chem.*, **42**, 689 (1994).
71. Y. Nishi, Y. Miyakawa and K. Kato, *Mut. Res.*, **227**, 117 (1989).
72. Y. Miyakaw, Y. Nishi, K. Kato, H. Sato, M. Takahashi and Y. Hayashi, *Carcinogenesis*, **12**, 1169 (1991).
73. H. U. Aeschbacher, Ch. Chappuis, M. Manganel and R. Aeshbach, *Prog. Food Nutr. Sci.*, **5**, 279 (1981).
74. W. D. Powrie, C. H. Wu, M. P. Rosin and H. F. Stich, *J. Food Sci.*, **46**, 1433 (1981).
75. A. M. Pearson, C. Chen, J. I. Gray and S. D. Aust, *Free Radicals Biol. Med.*, **13**, 161 (1992).
76. F. Jaccaud and H. U. Aeschbacher, in *The Maillard Reaction in Food Processing, Human Nutrition, and Physiology* (eds. P. A. Finot, H. U. Aeschbacher, F. R. Hurrell and R. Liardon), Birkhäuser Verlag, Basel, 1990.
77. M. K. Shigenaga, C. J. Gimeno and B. N. Ames, *Proc. Natl Acad. Sci. (USA)*, **86**, 9697 (1989).
78. R. E. Cathcart, R. L. Schwiers, S. Ames and B. N. Ames, *Proc. Natl Acad. Sci. (USA)*, **81**, 5633 (1984).
79. R.Teoule, *Int. J. Radiat. Biol.*, **51**, 573 (1987).
80. L. Szilard, *Proc. Natl Acad. Sci. (USA)*, **45**, 30 (1959).
81. M. Meuth, *Biochim. Biophys. Acta*, **1032**, 1 (1990).
82. T. Lindahl and B. Nyberg, *Biochem.*, **11**, 3610 (1972).
83. T. Lindahl and A. Andersson, *Biochem.*, **11**, 3619 61972).
84. E. C. Friedberg, in *DNA Repair*, Freeman and Company, New York (1985).
85. R. G. Dean and R. G. Cutler, *Exp. Gerontol.*, **13**, 287 (1978).
86. R. R. Tice, in *Aging and DNA-Repair Capability* (ed. E. Schneider), Plenum Press, New York, 1978.
87. H. R. Warner and A. R. Price, *J. Gerontol.*, **44**, 45 (1989).
88. Y. Fujiwara, M. Tatsumi and M. S. Sasaki, *J. Mol. Biol.*, **113**, 635 (1977).
89. F. Marlhens, W. A. Achkar, A. Aurias, J. Couturier, A. M. Dutrillaux, M. Gerbault-Sereau, F. Hoffschir, E. Lamoliatte, D. Lefrancois, M. Lombard, M. Muleris, M. Prieur, M. Prod'homme, L. Sabatier, E. Vieges-Pequignot, V. Volobouev and B. Dutrillaux, *Hum. Genet.*, **73**, 290 (1986).
90. M. Prieur, W. A. Achkar, A. Auriar, J. Couturier, A. M. Dutrillaux, B. Dutrillaux, A. Flury-Herard, M. Gerbault-Sereau, F. Hoffschir, E. Lamoliatte, D. Lefrancois, M. Lombard, M. Muleris, M. Ricoul, L. Sabatier and E. Vieges-Pequignot, *Hum. Genet.*, **79**, 147 (1988).
91. E. Solomon, J. Borrow and A. D. Goddard, *Science*, **254**, 1153 (1991).
92. Y. Liu, A. M. Hernandez, D. Shibata and G. A. Cortopassi, *Proc. Natl Acad. Sci. (USA)*, **91**, 8910 (1994).
93. P. Ebbesen, *Mech. Age Devel.*, **25**, 269 (1984).
94. M. C. Pike, M. D. Krailo, B. E. Henderson, J. T. Casagrande and D. G. Hoel, *Nature*, **303**, 767 (1983).
95. R. B. Setlow, in *DNA Repair among Humans* (eds. C. C. Harris and H. N. Autrup), Academic Press, London, 1983.

96. N. P. Singh, D. B. Danner, R. R. Tice, L. Brant and E. L. Schneider, *Mutation Res.*, **237**, 123 (1990).
97. A. T. Lee, C. DiSimone, A. Cerami and R. Bucala, *FASEB J.*, **8**, 545 (1994).
98. A. T. Lee, A. Plump, C. DiSimone, A. Cerami and R. Bucala, *Diabetes*, **44**, 20 (1995).
99. J. L. Mills, *Teratology*, **25**, 385 (1982).
100. L. Cousina, *Am. J. Obstet. Gynecol.*, **147**, 333 (1983).

9

Maillard Reaction under Microwave Irradiation

VAROUJAN A. YAYLAYAN

Department of Food Science and Agricultural Chemistry,
McGill University, Quebec, Canada

INTRODUCTION

Flavors and colors generated as a result of the Maillard reaction are of critical importance for the commercial success of microwave processed foods. Recent interest in the microwave generation of Maillard aromas and colors was a response on the part of the food industry for commercial exploitation of the consumer demand for fast and convenient food products. However, food products heated under microwave irradiation lack the color and flavor associated with the Maillard reaction observed under conventional heating (McGorrin et al., 1994). The fundamental differences between microwave and conventional heating, the composition of the food matrix and the design of microwave ovens all seem to play a role in the inability of microwave heating to propagate Maillard reactions in food products to generate desirable color and aroma. The increased penetration, in the last decade, of microwave ovens, especially into the North American market, provided the food industry with the impetus for renewed interest in carrying out the Maillard reaction in food products, under microwave irradiation.

Application of microwave energy to carry out chemical reactions has gained considerable importance in the late 1980s after the discovery that a wide range of reactions can be completed under microwave irradiation in a much shorter period of time compared to conventional heating by reflux (Gedye et al., 1986, 1988, 1991). Microwave heating can be effected by microwave energy

The Maillard Reaction: Consequences for the Chemical and Life Sciences. Edited by Raphael Ikan
©1996 John Wiley & Sons Ltd

(frequency range of $300–3.0 \times 10^5$ MHz) while conventional heating by conduction, convection or radiant energy (frequency range of 3.0×10^5–3.0×10^8 MHz, infrared region). Both are electromagnetic radiations with differing frequencies and hence wavelengths. Most domestic microwave ovens use the 2450 ± 13 MHz frequency with a wavelength of 12.2 cm and an energy output of 600–700 W. Radiant energy has a wavelength in the range of 1–10 μm (Peterson, 1993). This difference in wavelengths has the most important consequence to microwave heating of food matrices and on the ensuing chemical reactions in terms of penetration depth and rate of heat transfer. Because of differences in wavelengths, microwave energy penetrates deeper according to the following equation (assuming that the dielectric properties of a matter remain the same over both frequency ranges, microwave energy can penetrate a thousand times deeper than infrared):

$$D_p = \frac{\lambda_0 \sqrt{\varepsilon'}}{2\pi\varepsilon''} \tag{1}$$

where D_p = depth at which the microwave power is 37% (or $1/e$) of its
         value at the surface level
         λ_0 = wavelength in air
         ε' = dielectric constant
         ε'' = dielectric loss factor

The dielectric loss factor (ε'') indicates the amount of input energy dissipated as heat. The ratio of $\varepsilon''/\varepsilon'$ is known as the dissipation factor (or tan δ) upon which depends the rate of absorption of microwave energy. The faster the microwaves are absorbed and dissipated into a sample the lower is its penetration (D_p) and hence the greater is the sample's dissipation factor. The rate at which temperature is increased when materials absorb microwave energy is given by

$$\text{Rate} = k \, \frac{\nu E^2 \varepsilon''}{\rho C_p} \tag{2}$$

where k = rate constant
         ν = frequency
         E = electrical field strength
         ρ = density of the material
         C_p = specific heat
         ε'' = dielectric loss factor

The conversion of microwave energy into heat can be achieved by two mechanisms: dipole rotation and ionic conduction; consequently only ionic and dipolar molecules can interact with microwaves to generate heat. The resistance due to the ionic migration under the applied electromagnetic field results in heat generation by ionic conduction. On the other hand, the heat released through dipole rotation refers to the alignment of molecules that have permanent or induced dipole moments with the electromagnetic field and their subsequent relaxation into thermally induced disorder as the field is removed and thermal energy is released. The process of dipole rotation occurs 4.9×10^9 times per second (at the frequency of domestic microwave ovens) which results in an increased rate of heat generation. The relative importance of these two mechanisms of heat transfer depends to a large extent on the temperature, due to its effect on ion mobility and characteristic dielectric relaxation times (Neas and Collins, 1988).

Because of the high penetration depth and direct deposition of power to the sample, without heating the transfer medium (air), microwave heating is relatively fast. This property initiated the initial investigation into carrying out chemical reactions under microwave irradiation (Giguere *et al.*, 1986). In certain cases chemical reactions were completed in a few seconds that otherwise would have taken hours. In addition to fast rates of heating, microwaves are also more selective; components with high dielectric constants can be heated selectively in a reaction mixture compared to conventional heating. This property has been used to enhance the extraction of essential oils from plants immersed in a microwave transparent solvent (Paré *et al.*, 1991).

Superheating of solvents is another phenomenon that accompanies microwave heating and helps accelerate chemical reactions. Superheatng refers to the increase in temperature of liquids above their boiling points while they remain completely in the liquid phase. For example, water boils under microwave heating at 105 °C and acetonitrile (*b.p.* 82 °C) at 120 °C. A chemical reaction carried out in an open vessel in acetonitrile under microwave irradiation will be accelerated by 14 times relative to conventional heating, assuming that the reaction rate doubles for every 10 °C rise in temperature (Peterson, 1993). When chemical reactions are carried out in closed containers under microwave irradiation, the maximum temperatures attainable are not limited to the temperature of the heating medium, as in conventional heating, but depend only on microwave power applied and the rate at which the sample can lose heat (Peterson, 1993). The extremely high temperatures attained in a closed container during microwave heating can generate extremely high pressures (especially if the reaction produces gaseous products) which can alter equilibrium product distribution according to Le Chatelier's principle (Peterson, 1993).

The two aspects of microwave irradiation that affect the propagation of the Maillard reaction in foods include the interaction of microwaves with the food matrix and its effect on the chemical reactions in general. Unlike solvent-mediated Maillard reactions, the food matrix imparts special consideration, due to selective absorption of microwaves by different food components, compartmentalization of reactants, presence of components with differing loss factors, mobility of reactants, moisture content and presence of ionic species. Solvent-mediated and 'in-matrix' Maillard reactions will be discussed separately.

EFFECT OF MICROWAVE IRRADIATION
ON CHEMICAL REACTIONS:
SOLVENT-MEDIATED MAILLARD REACTIONS

The rates of chemical reactions depend primarily on temperature, presure, time and concentration of reactants. High temperature, pressure and superheating of reaction solvent associated with microwave irradiation can accelerate simple or single-step chemical reactions such as esterification, hydrolysis, cyclization, Diels–Alder and S_N2-type reactions (Giguere *et al.*, 1986; Gedye *et al.*, 1988, Abramovich *et al.*, 1991; Banik *et al.*, 1992; Bose *et al.*, 1994). If the microwave heating is done under a closed system, then the rate of the microwave reaction becomes even faster, up to one thousand times. For example, the per cent yield of 1-propyl benzoate after heating equal amounts of reactants for 4 min in an oil bath at 160 °C and in the microwave oven in an open vessel for 4 min was identical within experimental errors. The same reaction produces a yield of 79% for 6 min of microwave heating in a closed system, compared to 4 h refluxing which produces the same yield. In a closed system microwave irradiation increases the rate of the esterification reaction by 40 times (Gedye *et al.*, 1988). However, the time factor plays a crucial role in influencing the product distribution of more complex reactions when carried out under microwave heating. One important consequence of the fast rate of heating under microwave irradiation that is specially pertinent to the propagation of the Maillard reaction is its influence on competitive and consecutive reactions. In the competitive (or parallel) reaction shown below, reactants A and B produce two products P_1 and P_2 by two separate mechanisms, such that P_1 is more stable than P_2 and the activation energy (E_{a2}) to produce P_2 is relatively smaller than that of P_1. The reaction mixture produced under microwave heating (fast increase in temperature) of A and B will be richer in P_1 compared to the conventionally heated (slow increase in temperature) sample for the same length of time. The reaction at the high temperature of the microwave will be under thermodynamic control and will produce the most stable product in higher yields (Bond *et al.*, 1992).

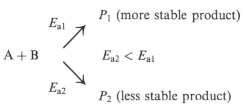

In the case of consecutive reactions of the type shown below, where the reaction produces color as the end product, the rate of formation of E from B will depend on the concentration of D and the rate of formation of D, in return, will depend on the concentration of C. Until there is considerable accumulation of C and D very little E will be formed.

$$B \longrightarrow C \longrightarrow D \longrightarrow E \longrightarrow \text{color}$$

Heating a solution of B under microwave irradiation will produce a mixture containing relatively less of C, D and E compared to a similar solution heated conventionally to reach the same temperature as in the microwave. If E is the precursor of a color-producing species, then the microwave-heated sample will reach the same temperature as the conventionally heated mixture in a shorter period of time with a lower yield of E and hence color. The Maillard reaction (Scheme 1), being such a complex series of consecutive and competitive reactions, will be most affected by microwave irradiation relative to conventional

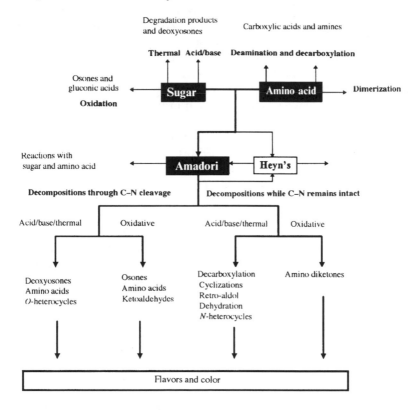

Scheme 1. Complex pathways of Maillard reaction

heating in terms of product distribution and intensity of browning. Generally, the final outcome of the Maillard reaction (color, volatile aroma compounds and nonvolatile products) depends on temperature, water content, pH and heating time; any variation in the reaction parameters will affect the profile of the end-products, and hence the perceived aroma and color.

Although simple chemical reactions are fast under microwave irradiation, multistep reactions can remain incomplete or they do not proceed to the same extent as under conventional heating, producing mixtures, although containing the same products (Yaylayan *et al.*, 1994) but with altered distribution patterns. The flavor perception is sensitive to such variations in relative concentrations of different components, especially the character impact compounds, thus drastically changing the sensory properties.

There are few reports in the literature on the microwave-assisted generation of Maillard products using precursors or intermediates. Preparative scale microwave-assisted synthesis (Chen *et al.*, 1990) of Amadori products from D-glucose and amino acids is feasible but has not been reported. However, Barbiroli *et al.* (1978) observed 70–75% conversion of added glucose–leucine into Amadori compound with a corresponding decrease in the amount of added amino acid in bread mix when microwaved for 3 min. Steinke *et al.* (1989) generated Strecker aldehydes from an aqueous solution of an amino acid and 2,3-butadione (diacetyl) in sealed vials microwaved for 4 minutes or heated in a water bath for 60 minutes at the same temperature. Significantly higher concentrations of aldehydes were measured in the microwave-heated samples. The effect of electrolytes and pH on the formation of Maillard products during microwave irradiation of aqueous model systems has been studied. The addition of different salts (Yeo and Shibamoto, 1991a), such as sodium chloride, calcium chloride and sodium sulfate, increased both the intensity of browning and the concentration of flavor compounds. The total volatiles generated from a glucose–cysteine model system (Yeo and Shibamoto, 1991b) under microwave irradiation has been found to increase with pH. It seems that increasing the pH and concentration of electrolytes enhances the rate of Maillard reactions under microwave irradiation. This observation, although consistent with the mechanism of heat generation by ionic conduction, might be influenced by the water activity changes associated with the addition of salts.

Attempts have been made to compare the chemical composition and yields of volatiles in microwaved and conventionally heated Maillard model systems. However, this type of comparison can be misleading due to the variations in the time–temperature exposure of the two systems under study. In most cases the temperature of the microwave system is not monitored and time of irradiation is chosen arbitrarily. In order to compare the yields of two systems undergoing the same reaction at different times and temperatures, a knowledge of kinetic parameters is required to ascertain whether there are differences in the two processes. Alternatively, the intensity of brown color formation can be used as an indication that the two systems have undergone equivalent time–temperature exposure. Yaylayan *et al.* (1994) subjected the same sugar–amino acid mixtures in water to microwave irradiation (640 W) and to conventional heating in an open system, until all the water was evaporated and the residue was dark brown, to mimic actual cooking conditions that require surface drying of foods. In order to insure that both treatments produced the same extent of Maillard reaction for comparison purposes, the conventional heating time was adjusted such that, after similar dilutions, both samples absorbed to the same extent at 460 nm in the spectrophotometer. On average, one minute of microwave heating time was equivalent to 12 minutes of conventional heating time to produce the same extent of browning. With such treatment no significant qualitative changes were observed in the composition of both samples identified by GC/MS (gas chromatography/mass spectrometry). Parliment (1993) studied, in sealed vials, the products of the Maillard reaction between glucose and proline formed under microwave (600 W, pre-heated conventionally for 3 min and irradiated for 45 s) and conventionally heated systems (150 °C for 15 min). Qualitatively both systems produced similar compounds but in the microwave system *N*-heterocyclic compounds were present in smaller amounts. These types of experiment are inconclusive since the temperature of the microwave sample is not measured to estimate whether heating at 150 °C for 15 min is equivalent to 45 s of microwave irradiation. Ji and Bernhard (1992), on the other hand, calculated the *pseudo* zero-order rate constants for selected pyrazines produced in mixtures consisting of D-glucose and glycine in 100 mL of water, microwaved (500 W) in an open system for between 1.5 and 9.0 minutes. The temperature of all the samples were measured after the completion of the irradiation and found to be around 100 °C. The calculated rate constants were found to be in agreement with those reported under conventional heating (Leahy and Reineccius, 1989). In addition, when the products of the microwave sample (9.0 min of irradiation at 100 °C) were compared with those produced under conventional heating at 120 °C for 4.0 h, the total yield of the products increased from 4.4 to 6.6% based on the D-glucose concentration. In general, the Maillard model studies indicate that there are no fundamental differences between microwave and conventionally heated samples in the solution phase except in time–temperature exposure of the two systems and hence in the relative amounts of products formed.

INTERACTION OF MICROWAVE IRRADIATION WITH THE FOOD MATRIX: THE MAILLARD REACTION IN FOOD PRODUCTS

At the molecular level, the mechanism of heat generation in the microwave oven relies mainly on the interaction of the microwave radiation with dipoles/

induced dipoles or with ions. Proteins and lipids do not significantly interact with microwave radiation in the presence of aqueous ions that selectively absorb the radiation because of their enhanced interaction with microwave radiation. However, in the absence of water, lipids and colloidal solids are known to interact strongly with microwave radiation; the observed levels of energy absorption cannot be explained by the presence of free water and by ion activity (Pomeranz and Meloan, 1987). Microwave radiation can also interact with alcohols, sugars and polysachharides. Tightly bound water monolayers do not absorb energy due to hindered molecular rotations. Overall, the extent of heat generation by microwave irradiation depends mainly on the moisture and salt content of food products.

Microwave interactions with a multicomponent system such as food can differ considerably from simple aqueous Maillard model systems, in that 'matrix effects' can produce undesirable consequences. Since the core aqueous regions of foods are the main sites of interaction with the microwaves, the interor vapor pressure generated as a result can actively force the vapor to the surface of the food, unlike in the conventional oven, where passive migration of water by capillary action to the surface is diffusion controlled (Schiffmann, 1994). The water-saturated food surfaces usually remain at relatively cool temperatures of the oven during cooking (40–60 °C), thus preventing browning and crisping (Schiffmann, 1994). Model studies have already indicated that there are no fundamental differences in the solution phase chemistry of the Maillard reaction under microwave irradiation. However, the overall performance of food products under microwave irradiation implies development of characteristic textural, color and aroma properties similar to that of conventional heating, which differs markedly from microwave heating due to the fast rate of heating and 'matrix effects'.

Food products that rely heavily on Maillard flavors and colors such as roasted and baked products perform well in the conventional oven due to:

1. The high temperature of the air surrounding the product, which dehydrates the surface, producing a crust that protects the food from loss of moisture and important aroma volatiles. Dehydration steps are also crucial for the formation of color and aroma precursors by the Maillard reaction.
2. Long-time exposure in the conventional oven ensures the completion of slow and/or multistep Maillard reactions responsible for browning and for the generation of specific aromas. In the microwave oven, the short-time exposure and the lack of hot dry air (air being transparent to microwave irradiation) surrounding the surface of the food product not only prevents crusting but also promotes sogginess due to the condensation of the moisture. On the other hand, the rapid release of moisture and its evaporation from, the center of the food causes the added and formed volatiles to be 'steam distilled' at temperatures below their boiling points.

Hence baked and roasted food products which rely heavily on Maillard produced flavors usually do not perform well in the microwave oven.

Schiffmann (1994) summarized the different factors related to microwave ovens that effect aroma generation during the cooking of food, such as the variation in the type of commercial oven (power, cavity size, etc.) and its effect on the reproducibility of performance, speed of heating, oven temperature and vapor pressure buildup inside the food. The short time required in the microwave oven to attain the same temperature as in the conventional oven not only retards the Maillard reaction but also prevents the establishment of thermal equilibrium throughout the food and uniform temperature distribution through conductive heat transfer, thus creating hot and cold spots in the food product which aggravates further the oven hot and cold zones created as a result of standing wave patterns. In addition, different dielectric loss factors (ε'') associated with different components in a multicomponent food product will also contribute to the uneven heating pattern inside the microwave oven. The combined effect of these phenomena is manifested in the excessive exposure of certain parts of the food to heat and diminished exposure in others, leading to undesirable textural and flavor modifications such as charring, drying, excessive evaporation, hardening and development of burnt or raw flavor and aroma notes. The extent of these undesirable modifications is dependent on the size, geometry, thickness and the composition of the food product (Schiffmann, 1994). Yeo and Shibamoto (1991c) reviewed the chemical composition of volatiles generated by microwave and conventionally heated food products. White cake batters were cooked to the same degree, both in the microwave and the conventional oven. The volatiles released and sensory properties of both products were compared (Whorton and Reineccius, 1989). The number of volatiles detected and the amount of total pyrazines produced were found to be more in the conventionally baked sample. In addition, the microwave cake lacked the nutty, caramel and brown-type flavors. In a similar study (MacLeod and Coppock, 1976), the number of volatiles generated from boiled beef cooked by microwave for one hour was found to be more than the number of volatiles generated by beef boiled conventionally for the same length of time. When both systems were compared on the basis of 'doneness', the microwave sample generated only one-third of the amount of volatiles detected in the conventional oven. The relative success of the microwave to achieve the Maillard effect of conventional heating may depend to a large degree on the type and composition of the food product.

Most of the model studies reported in the literature compare the volatiles generated by the Maillard reaction under microwave or conventional heating to elucidate the differences between the two modes of heating. However, in an interesting study, Barbiroli *et al.* (1978) compared the changes in the concentration of the added amino acids, amino acid–glucose mixtures and

Amadori rearrangement products (ARPs) in bread and biscuits baked by both methods. This approach provides more direct evidence of the differences in the chemical behaviour of sugar–amino acid mixtures in food matrices, when exposed to different modes of heating, than the analysis of volatiles. Table 9.1 summarizes the changes observed in the content of amino acids and ARPs in bread and biscuits after baking by microwave (3 minutes) and conventional ovens (220 °C for 30 minutes). In the conventional oven, most of the *in situ* formed ARPs from added sugar–amino acid mixtures were decomposed, whereas in the microwave oven, the ARPs accumulated instead. Model studies (Huyghues-Despointe and Yaylayan, 1994) have indicated that before any significant decomposition of ARP is initiated during the Maillard reaction, the concentration of Amadori product should reach a minimum value, and it seems under the experimental conditions that this was attained after 3 minutes. Microwaving the samples beyond the 3 minutes would have initiated the decomposition process. When Amadori compounds were added to biscuits, they decomposed more or less to the same extent during both types of heating, whereas in the case of bread, the decomposition of Amadori products under microwave heating was greater. The relative amounts of formation or decomposition, however, was dependent on the type of ARP and the food matrix. In the biscuit, for example, the decomposition of ARPs in the conventional oven is more pronounced than in the bread. This could be related to the differences in water content between bread (0.48 mL of water/g of solids)

Table 9.1. Percent loss of added amino acids and Amadori products and percent accumulation of Amadori products in bread and biscuits baked conventionally (bread: 220 °C for 30 min; biscuit: 240 °C for 20 min) and under microwave (3 min). (Adapted from Barbiroli *et al.*, 1978)

Added components	Conventional oven		Microwave oven	
	Amino acid (bread/biscuit)	ARP* (bread/biscuit)	Amino acid (bread/biscuit)	ARP* (bread/biscuit)
Leucine	−3%/−19%		−15%/−15%	
Leucine + glucose	−6%/−25%	+8%/+3%	−95%/−53%	+66%/+71%
Leucine ARP	trace/+32%	−14%/−92%	+30%/+36%	−97%/−93%
Valine	−6%/−8%		−3%/−3%	
Valine + glucose	−6%/−15%	+0%/+6%	−68%/−60%	+97%/+82%
Valine ARP	+9%/+33%	−22%/−80%	+40%/+37%	−96%/−88%

*Percent weight formation relative to glucose
ARP: Amadori rearrangement product
− loss
+ Formation of ARP or release of amino acid from ARP

and biscuit (0.34 mL of water/g of solids) and the temperature of baking. Interestingly, in the microwave oven the amounts of both the accumulated and decomposed ARPs were not dependent significantly on the type of food matrix.

The result of this study clearly shows that the Amadori product, the main precursor of Maillard aromas and colors, can be formed from sugar and amino acids found in food under microwave heating (3 min), but does not decompose efficiently during the short time-scale of microwave exposure.

DEVELOPMENT OF NEW PRODUCTS/PROCESSES TO OVERCOME LIMITATIONS OF MICROWAVE HEATING IN PROPAGATING MAILLARD REACTION IN FOOD SYSTEMS

In the last decade, the sales of microwave food products have experienced a larger growth rate compared to overall food sales due to the convenience offered by such products to the consumers. As a result, food products specifically formulated to perform under microwave irradiation have become priority areas of research in many food companies (Decareau, 1992). This trend, however, seems to be changing (Sloan, 1994) as the number of domestic microwave ovens used in functions other than heating has fallen from almost 45% in the mid 1980s to under 30% in the early 1990s (Balzer, 1993). The sales projection for microwave-only food products of $4 billion for 1997 may reach only $2.7 billion from today's $2.4 billion market (Find/SVP, 1993).

Different strategies have been attempted to overcome the lack of Maillard flavor and color development during microwaving. Some were aimed at packaging technologies, others at the modifications of food and flavor formulations or addition to food of specific formulations containing Maillard-active ingredients to promote flavor and/or color development. One of the earliest attempts by the food industry to promote surface browning in foods formulated for microwave irradiation was the use of susceptor packaging. Susceptors are metalized polyethylene teraphthalate (PET) films laminated on paperboards, which can interact with electromagnetic radiation and generate localized heating near the surface of foods, when incorporated with the packaging materials of microwave food products (Shaath and Azzo, 1990). While susceptors are effective in promoting surface browning, they do not allow the full development of flavors (Reineccius and Whorton, 1990).

Designing flavor formulations containing components with reduced volatility to prevent their loss is based on the concept of selective volatilization under microwave heating. Although the rate of microwave heating of individual components in a food depends on their dielectric constants and loss factors, such that compounds having similar specific heats but high loss factors heat more rapidly under microwave irradiation, however, their rate of volatilization from the food matrix depends on the overall temperature of the food (Lindstrom and Parliment, 1994) and on the chemical interactions with the environment and their solubility properties (Stanford and McGorrin, 1994; Steinke *et al.*, 1989). These factors should be taken into consideration when flavor formulations are modified for microwave applications.

Shaath and Azzo (1989) proposed what they termed 'Delta T' theory' as a basis to design microwave stable flavor formulations. This hypothesis is based on experimentally obtained $\Delta T'$ values for individual flavor compounds used frequently in flavor formulations. These values indicate the increase in temperature of a solution of a pure flavor compound relative to an equivalent amount of water when similarly exposed to microwave irradiation. $\Delta T'$ values have been found to increase with dielectric constant (ε') values in a series of compounds having the same specific heat. Shaath and Azzo (1989) claim that selecting flavor compounds for microwave formulations with values less than that of water ($\Delta T' = 1$) will prevent their volatilization during microwaving 'Delta T' theory' has been justifiably criticized for not taking into consideration the effect of food matrix interactions with the flavor compounds (Reineccius and Whorton, 1990) and for its inability to predict the microwave behavior of a mixture of flavor compounds (Schwarzenbach, 1990). Experimental evidence (Graf and de Roos, 1994) indicates that the temperature of individual flavor compounds in food cannot be significantly different from the bulk temperature of the food matrix since the heat generated by individual compounds is dissipated quickly into the surrounding medium with no significant influence on the overall temperature due to their low concentrations. In addition, Steinke *et al.* (1989) have demonstrated the solvent (matrix) dependence of microwave volatilization of aromas. Therefore, $\Delta T'$ values relative to water may not be used to predict the microwave behavior of flavor mixtures in complex food systems.

Graf and de Roos (1994), on the other hand, developed a mathematical model that takes into account the food matrix interactions and compartmentalization of aroma compounds in addition to their volatility and hydrophobicity to predict the behavior of a flavor mixture under microwave irradiation. The model considers the food matrix as an oil/water emulsion and the process of volatilization of aroma as a repeated water extraction step. The fraction (f) of flavor compounds remaining in an oil/water emulsion after equilibration with air in a closed system was calculated by

$$f = \frac{V_w P_{ao} + V_o P_{aw}}{V_a P_{aw} P_{ao} + V_w P_{ao} + V_o P_{aw}} \tag{3}$$

where $\quad V_w$ = volume of water (mL)
$\qquad\ P_{ao}$ = air to oil partition coefficient
$\qquad\ V_o$ = volume of oil (mL)

V_a = volume of air

P_{aw} = air to water partition coefficient

The validity of this equation to predict the equilibrium concentrations of food volatiles was demonstrated in a model study using milk with five added aroma compounds. The experimentally determined concentrations of milk headspace volatiles were in good agreement with the calculated values using Eqn (3). The static equilibrium equation shown above was transformed into an equation that describes dynamic nonequilibrium systems characteristic of foods during microwave heating. This transformation was based on the assumption that foods under microwave heating undergo consecutive extractions with infinitesimal volumes of moisture. The fraction (f_n) of flavor compounds remaining in the food after n number of extraction cycles is given by

$$f_n = [1 - f_e + f_e(f)]^n \tag{4}$$

where f_e = fraction of food being extracted

   n = number of successive extractions

   f = giver by Eqn (3)

Equation (4) successfully predicted, with an overall correlation coefficient of 0.96, the flavor release from microwave cake samples. In general, the model demonstrates that the rate of aroma volatilization is determined by the partition coefficients of flavor compounds, chemical physical properties of food matrix, moisture loss and amount of heat input. Although modifications of flavor formulations based on such mathematical models might reduce the loss of added flavors by volatilization, they do not address the problem of Maillard flavor and color generation during microwaving.

As has been implicated in the previous sections, the failure of microwave heating to develop flavors and colors is due to the limited time-scale of microwave exposure of foods to elevated temperatures necessary to carry out the Maillard reaction. The main strategy used to overcome this limitation is the addition of reactive Maillard reaction precursors to the surface of foods to accelerate the Maillard reaction such that it can be accomplished within the short time frame of microwave cooking (10–15 minutes). Most of the patent literature, however, discloses processes to generate browning rather than specific aromas and browning. The general requirement for microwave-reactive Maillard mixtures is their ability to generate, in addition to color, either no aroma or an aroma that is compatible with the intended product. Browning-only precursors could have a wider range of applications in different food products. The general composition of such mixtures reported in the patent literature includes reactive sugars and amino acids/protein hydrolysates in addition to a promoter (an alkaline component). These mixtures could be applied to the surface of foods either as liquids or as dried powders; alternatively reactants could be encapsulated in a carrier. Bryson *et al.* (US Pat. 4,735,812 issued on 5 April 1988) developed a browning agent composed of hydrolyzed collagen or gelatin mixed with reducing sugars and a mixture of sodium carbonate and bicarbonate. The browning agent could be applied on the surface of foods to be microwaved either as a powder or as a liquid. Parliment *et al.* (US Pat. 4,857,340 issued on 15 August 1989) describe an aroma-producing precursor encapsulated in a lipid carrier capable of releasing aroma under microwave irradiation when placed in close proximity to a microwave-susceptible material. Kang *et al.* (US Pat. 5,059,434 issued on 22 October 1991) disclose a process for manufacturing a browning powder for muscle foods composed of separately encapsulated reactive sugars (xylose, arabinose, etc.), amino acids (lysine, arginine, etc.) or hydrolyzed vegetable proteins and a Maillard reaction promoter (polyvinyl pyrolidone). A similar patent (US Pat. 5,091,200 issued on 25 February 1992) for baked goods was also issued to the same inventors. Steinke *et al.* (US Pat. 5,043,173 issued on 27 August 1991) describe a browning water-in-oil emulsion containing only a reactive carbonyl compound and an edible hydrophilic base such that, upon heating, the emulsion breaks down and brings the reactants together to initiate browning during microwave heating. Yaylayan *et al.* (1994) reported on the development of microwave-active Maillard formulations that can generate browning and at the same time deliver specific aromas (baked, roasted, chicken, beef, etc.) when coated on targeted food products. To facilitate the choice of amino acids in these mixtures, the potential of different amino acids to produce specific aroma notes in the microwave was evaluated.

The fact that at present there are no successful microwave-specific food products attests to the failure of the current strategies to solve the problem. These strategies, aimed at the modification of the food product to conform to the environment of microwave ovens, perhaps should be redirected into modification of the microwave oven design to conform to the specific nature of the food matrix.

REFERENCES

Abramovitch, R. A., Abramovitch, D. A., Iyanar, K., and Tamareselvy, K. (1991). Application of microwave energy to organic synthesis: improved technology, *Tetrahedron Lett.*, **32**, 5251–4.

Balzer, H. (1993). The ultimate cooking appliance. *Am. Demographics*, **July**, 40–4.

Banik, B. K., Manhas, M. S., Kaluza, Z., Barakat, K. J., and Bose, A. K. (1992). Microwave-induced organic reaction enhancement chemistry. 4. Convenient synthesis of enantiopure α-hydroxy-β-lactams, *Tetrahedron Lett.*, **33**, 3603–6.

Barbiroli, G., Garutti, A. M., and Mazzaracchio, P. (1978). Note on behavior of 1-amino-1-deoxy-2-ketose derivatives during cooking when added to starch based foodstuffs, *Cereal Chem.*, **55**, 1056–9.

Bond, S. P., Hall, C. E., McNerlin, C. J., and McWhinnie, W. R. J. (1992). Coordination compounds on the surface of laponite-tri-pyridylamine complexes, *Mater. Chem.*, **2**, 37.

Bose, A. K., Manhas, M. S., Banik, B. K., and Robb, E. W. (1994). Microwave-induced organic reaction enhancement. (MORE) chemistry: techniques for rapid, safe and inexpensive synthesis, *Res. Chem. Intermed.*, **20**, 1–11.

Chen, S. T., Chiou, S. H., and Wang, K. T. (1990). Preparative scale organic synthesis using a kitchen microwave oven, *J. Chem. Soc., Chem. Commun.*, **11**, 807–9.

Decareau, R. V. (1992). *Microwave Foods: New Product Development*, Food and Nutrition Press Inc., Trumbell, Connecticut.

Find/SVP (1993). *The Market of Microwavable Foods*, Find/SVP, New York.

Gedye, R., Smith, F., Westaway, K., Ali, H., Baldisera, L., Laberge, L., and Rousell, J. (1986). The use of microwave ovens for rapid organic synthesis, *Tetrahedron Lett.*, **27**, 279–82.

Gedye, R. N., Smith, F. E., and Westaway, K. C. (1988). The rapid synthesis of organic compounds in microwave ovens, *Can. J. Chem.*, **66**, 17–26.

Gedye, R. N., Rank, W., and Westaway, K. C. (1991). The rapid synthesis of organic compounds in microwave ovens. II. *Can. J. Chem.*, **69**, 706–11.

Giguere, R. J., Bray, T. L., Duncan, S. M., and Majetich, G. (1986). Application of commercial microwave ovens to organic synthesis, *Tetrahedron Lett.*, **27**, 4945–8.

Graf, E., and de Roos, K. (1994). Nonequilibrium partition model for prediction of microwave flavor release. In J. McGorrin, T. H. Parliment and M. J. Morello (eds.), *Thermally generated flavors: Maillard, Microwave and Extrusion Processes*, ACS Symposium Series 543, American Chemical Society, Washington, D.C., pp. 437–48.

Huyghues-Despointe, A., and Yaylayan, V. (1994). Kinetics of formation and degradation of morpholino-1-deoxy-D-fructose. In C.-H. Tong, C.-T. Tan and C.-T. Ho (eds.), *Flavor Technology*, ACS Symposium Series, No. 610, American Chemical Society, Washington, D.C. (in press).

Ji, H., and Bernhard, R. A. (1992) Effect of microwave heating on pyrazine formation in a model system, *J. Sci. Food Agric.*, **59**, 283–9.

Leahy, M. M., and Reineccius, G. A. (1989). Kinetics of formation of alkylpyrazines-effect of type of amino acid and type of sugar. In R. Teranishi, R. G. Buttery and F. Shahidi (eds.), *Flavor chemistry: trends and developments*, ACS Symposium Series 388, American Chemical Society, Washington, D.C., pp. 76–91.

Lindstrom, T. R., and Parliment, T. H. (1994). Microwave volatilization of aroma compounds. In J. McGorrin, T. H. Parliment and M. J. Morello (eds.), *Thermally Generated Flavors: Maillard, Microwave and Extrusion Processes*, ACS Symposium Series 543, American Chemical Society, Washington, D.C., pp. 405–13.

McGorrin, J., Parliment, T. H., and Morello, M. J. (eds.) *Thermally Generated Flavors: Maillard, Microwave and Extensive Processes*, ACS Symposium Series 543, American Chemical Society, Washington, D.C.

MacLeod, G. and Coppock, B. M. J. (1976). Volatile flavor components of beef boiled conventionally and by microwave radiation, *Agric. Food Chem.*, **24**, 835–43.

Neas, E. D., and Collins, M. J. (1988). Microwave heating. In H. M. Kingston and L. B. Jassie (eds.), *Introduction to Microwave Sample Preparation: Theory and Practice*, American Chemical Society, Washington, D.C., pp. 7–32.

Paré, J. R., Sigouin, M., and Lapointe, J. (1991). US Pat. 5,002,784, issued on 26 March 1991.

Parliment, T. H. (1993). Comparison of thermal and microwave mediated Maillard reactions. In G. Charalambous (ed.), *Food Flavors, Ingredients and Composition*, Elsevier, Amsterdam, pp. 657–62.

Peterson, E. R. (1993). Microwave chemistry: a conceptual review of the literature. In *Quality Enhancement Using Microwaves*, 28th Annual Microwave Symposium Proceedings, International Microwave Power Institute.

Pomeranz, Y., and Meloan, C. E. (1987). *Food Analysis: Theory and Practice*, 2nd ed., Van Reinhold Nostrand Co., New York.

Reineccius, G., and Whorton, C. (1990). Flavor problems associated with the microwave cooking of food products. In P. Finot, H. Aeschbacher, R. F. Hurrell and R. Liardon (eds.), *The Maillard Reaction in Food Processing, Human Nutrition and Physiology*, Birkhäuser, Basel, p. 197.

Schiffmann, R. F. (1994). Critical factors in microwave-generated aromas. In J. McGorrin, T. H. Parliment and M. J. Morello (eds.), *Thermally Generated Flavors: Maillard, Microwave and Extrusion Processes*, ACS Symposium Series 543, American Chemical Society, Washington, D. C., pp. 386–94.

Schwarzenbach, R. (1990). Microwave stable flavors — development or promotion? In *Flavor Science and Technology*, John Wiley & Sons, Chichester, pp. 281–96.

Shaath, N. A., and Azzo, N. R. (1989). In T. Parliment, R. McGorrin and C.-T. Ho (eds.), *Thermal Generation of Aromas*, ACS Symposium Series 409, American Chemical Society, Washington, D.C., p. 512.

Shaath, N. A., and Azzo, N. R. (1990). Latest developments in microwavable food and flavor formulations. In G. Charalambous (ed.), *Flavors and Off-Flavors*, Elsevier Science Publishers, Amsterdam, pp. 671–86.

Sloan, A. E. (1994). Top ten trends to watch and work on, *Food Technol.*, **48**, 96.

Stanford, A., and McGorrin, J. (1994). Flavor volatilization in microwave food model systems. In J. McGorrin, T. H. Parliment and M. J. Morello (eds.), *Thermally Generated Flavors: Maillard, Microwave and Extrusion Processes*, ACS Symposium Series 543, American Chemical Society, Washington, D.C., pp. 414–36.

Steinke, J. A., Frick, C. M., Gallagher, J. A., and Strassburger, K. J. (1989). Influence of microwave heating on flavor. In T. Parliment, R. McGorrin and C.-T. Ho (eds.), *Thermal General of Aromas*, ACS Symposium Series 409, American Chemical Society, Washington, D.C., pp. 520–5.

Whorton, C., and Reineccius, G. (1989). Flavor development in a microwaved versus a conventionally baked cake. In T. Parliment, R. McGorrin and C.-T. Ho (eds.), *Thermal Generation of Aromas*, ACS Symposium Series 409, American Chemical Society, Washington, D.C., p. 526.

Yaylayan, V., Forage, N. G., and Mandeville, S. (1994). Microwave and thermally induced Maillard reactions. In J. McGorrin, T. H. Parliment and M. J. Morello (eds.), *Thermally Generated Flavors: Maillard, Microwave and Extrusion Processes*, ACS Symposium Series 543, American Chemical Society, Washington, D.C., pp. 449–56.

Yeo, H. C. H., and Shibamoto, T. J. (1991a). Flavor and browning enhancement by electrolytes during microwave irradiation of the Maillard model systems, *Agric. Food Chem.*, **39**, 948–51.

Yeo, H. C. H., and Shibamoto, T. J. (1991b). Microwave-induced volatiles of the Maillard model system under different pH conditions, *Agric. Food Chem.*, **39**, 370–3.

Yeo, H. C. H., and Shibamoto, T. (1991c). Chemical comparison of flavours in microwaved and conventionally heated foods, *Trends Food Sci. Technol.*, **12**, 329.

Author Index

Subject Index